Shattered

MAVIS MARSH WITH ANDREW CROFTS

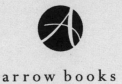

arrow books

This edition published 2008 for Index Books Ltd

10

This book is a work of non-fiction based on the life, experiences
and recollections of Mavis Marsh. In some limited cases names of people, places,
dates, sequences or the detail of events have been changed to protect the privacy of others.
The author has warranted to the publishers that, except in such minor respects not
affecting the substantial accuracy of the work, the contents of this book are true.
Whilst the publishers have taken care to explore and check where reasonably possible,
they have not verified all the information in this book and do not warrant its
veracity in all respects.

Arrow Books
The Random House Group Limited,
20 Vauxhall Bridge Road,
London SW1V 2SA

www.rbooks.co.uk

Addresses for companies within The Random House Group Limited can be found at:
www.randomhouse.co.uk/offices.htm

The Random House Group Limited Reg. No. 954009

A CIP catalogue record for this book
is available from the British Library

ISBN 9780099498513

The Random House Group Limited makes every effort to ensure that the papers used in its
books are made from trees that have been legally sourced from well-managed and credibly
certified forests. Our paper procurement policy can be found at:
www.rbooks.co.uk/environment

Typeset in Ehrhardt by Palimpsest Book Production Limited,
Kemfine, Earls Road, Grangemouth, Stirling FK3 8XG

Printed in the UK by CPI Bookmarque, Croydon, CR0 4TD

Contents

My thanks are only to Keith and Matthew for having the will to work so hard over the past 10 years.

Prologue

'Your son will be a cabbage for the rest of his life,' the senior doctor told us, 'or a vegetable, or whatever you want to call him.'

I almost gasped out loud at the cruel, callous words. They sounded to me like something a doctor fifty years ago would have said. A cabbage? A vegetable? Did they still refer to people like that?

My husband Keith and I sat and stared at the doctor and the head nurse from intensive care beside him. We were speechless. We couldn't believe what we were hearing.

Only a few hours before, our brilliant, popular, beautiful son was doing well. He was going to get better, his problems were minor. Under the circumstances, considering the terrible damage inflicted on his body, everything was as good as it could be.

Now the doctor was telling us that had all been a dream. Matthew wasn't going to get better after all. In fact, his future was nothing. It was a big blank canvas that would never be painted on. What had suddenly changed? Why were all the medical diagnoses, all the professional opinions, all the hope and optimism they had been feeding us with — gone, just like that? We couldn't take it in.

Through my shock it was hard to absorb what he said next, but I realised that in his strangely matter-of-fact way, the doctor was telling us to walk away from Matthew and get on with our lives. There was nothing we could do, he would never change. There was no hope.

Walk away? From our darling son, who lay helpless in a hospital bed just yards away? Were we supposed to stop thinking of him as Matthew, our wonderful son, and shrug our shoulders and say,

'Oh well, that's that, then. It's just a cabbage now,' and leave him?

Even at that moment, when Keith and I were both so deeply shocked and unable to take in what was happening, I don't think we ever believed for a second there was any possibility we could ever just walk away from Matthew, or from any of our children. It simply wasn't feasible. No matter what Matthew's future was, we would be there with him, for as long as he needed us.

We had no idea how we would care for our son, or what it would mean to us or to him. But we knew instinctively that there was no other choice. We couldn't just abandon him to the care of strangers, not when he was so helpless and vulnerable and unable to protect himself. It would be like giving away a newborn baby, even if he was twenty-five years old. I think almost any parent will understand that feeling.

When your children grow up, you know you have to let them go and live their lives independently; you want them to do that and you have years to grow used to the idea as the moment approaches. It is part of the natural process as each generation takes over from the one before.

But when one of your children suddenly returns to being as helpless as a baby, all the parental instincts that you had learned over the years to adapt and suppress come bubbling to the surface.

Matthew needed us, and he needed us desperately. We both knew that we were the only people who could help. Putting him in a home would condemn him to a twilight life, a nothing existence among people who didn't care for him. We felt that instinctively.

No. We'd never lock him away and forget about him.

The only trouble was that we had no idea what we would do instead.

1

War Baby

When you lose your memory you lose your whole sense of identity. I've had a lot of time to think about that over the last ten or so years, and to be grateful for the memories I have of my own past. Your memory tells you about who you are and where you've come from. It treasures the happiest recollections of your life: falling in love, wedding days, family parties, births, special journeys and good times with friends. It makes you laugh when you recall jokes or silly incidents; it can move you to tears when it conjures up the sad times, the bad days and the misery life can bring. It keeps the dead alive in our minds, it gives us our knowledge and the pleasure of our education. Our memories are fundamental to us all.

Imagine having nothing to look back on, no way of picturing who you were and how you became what you are today. Imagine knowing who your family are, but not remembering a single day you've spent with them. Imagine being told that you went to university, studied for a degree and travelled the world – but remembering absolutely nothing about it. That is surely a terrible fate. And that is what has happened to my son, Matthew.

My mum and dad moved to a council house in Middleton when I was a year old, in 1941. It was a nice three-bedroom house with a garden, indoor plumbing and hot water. Despite all the horrors that were going on at that time, as the Second World War raged across Europe and the Far East, our family wasn't doing too badly at all by the standards of the day.

Mum was a presser in a clothing factory. Before

she had children, she had been a bar lady, living in a public house. Dad worked on the bins. He would be called something much grander, like a 'refuse collector' now, but then he was just a binman and perfectly contented with his lot in life as far as anyone else could tell. He didn't drink or gamble or have any of the vices that so often led to hardship in other families we knew. They both took their pleasure in their family, working hard to make sure their children all got the best lives they could afford to give us.

It always made me feel special to be born when I was, because when we went into school people talked about us as 'the war babies', as if we already had a place in the history books alongside Winston Churchill, Spitfires and VE Day. Even though I was a war baby, I can't remember anything about the war itself at all. My oldest sister, Patricia, says she can remember hearing the doodlebugs coming over, but I can't. Like most people, the earliest part of my life didn't imprint itself on any part of my memory that I can find, and I can only recall what I was told later about the war, or saw in films. We did have a bomb shelter in the garden, which the council said we could buy off them once the danger of bombs had passed, but I don't remember ever having to use it for real. I think I was just too young for any of it to make an impression on my little world.

By the time I was old enough to be able to take anything in, the war was over. Hitler had been defeated and there was an air of optimism around, despite the lack of money and produce in the shops. None of us youngsters could remember a time of plenty anyway, so what difference did it make that there was a shortage of sugar or anything else? We had all we needed, we had survived and we had defeated the enemy. Nobody wanted to think about the past and all the bleak days of fighting and suffering, we were all eager to press on and the future looked bright.

We believed that now the war was won and we had the welfare state to help us get started, people like us could improve our lives and do whatever we wanted as long as we worked hard at school and didn't get ourselves into any trouble. Young people didn't feel they had to rebel in those days, not like they do now. As far as parents were concerned, the worst that could befall the girls was that they would get pregnant before marriage and for the boys the worst fear was that they would get on the wrong side of the law by doing something stupid. No one knew anything about illegal drugs, and they wouldn't have had the money to buy them even if they did. There wasn't much thieving because no one really had much worth stealing. All that was still to come.

I was the youngest of three sisters, following behind Patricia and Sheila. Mum was thirty-eight when I was born and Dad was forty-two. He had been too old to be called up to the army this time round; he had done his fighting in the First World War, although he never talked about it. He actually wanted to forget that part of his life, but I doubt he ever really did. The only thing he ever told us was that he was once in a forest in France, lying in a ditch while some Germans were passing by on the path above his head. He said he never believed it when he saw films about the war and the actors pretended not to be scared.

'I was so frightened,' he said, 'I actually messed myself.'

It was hard for me to imagine anything being so dreadful that a grown-up as strong as my dad was to me could be reduced to such a state of terror, but it all seemed a long way away, safely wrapped up in another time and another country.

He had still only been a teenager when he was shipped out to France and after the experiences he'd had there, he never wanted to leave England again, not even for a holiday. That didn't make him that unusual at the time; package holidays to Spain didn't really start coming in until the 1960s. Only the very rich got to go abroad, unless the forces sent them, and people like us took our holidays in such places as Blackpool or Scarborough. No one had the sort of money needed to buy a plane ticket.

'I've been abroad and seen it,' Dad would say later when travelling became cheaper and people began to sing the praises of overseas holidays. 'And I don't want to leave my country again.'

There is a lot to be said for being contented with your lot in life, and my dad was very contented.

Our house was on a lane, with a big garden both front and back, and was the last house on a great, sprawling estate. Opposite was a row of large private houses and behind them a small wood. At the end of the lane, open fields stretched all the way to Rothwell. At the other end were the local shops: a grocer, butcher and a fish-and-chip shop. When I got older I would babysit for the woman at the fish-and-chip shop while she and her husband served customers. They had a television and they always gave me a wonderful fish-and-chip dinner, as well as paying me for my time – so as you can imagine, I loved it there.

On my first day at school I met Rita, who became my first best friend, and we are still friends to this day, part of a tight little group who have been intimately involved in one another's lives now for over half a century. It's wonderful to have friends who remember everything about me, and who have experienced every stage of life with me, and that's not unusual in my generation. Although we might travel abroad on holiday more than our parents' generation, none of us have ever wanted to move away from the Middleton area and the people we've known all our lives. It would be the next generation, our children, who would start leaving.

Pat, who was four years older than me, was the

clever one of the family and at the age of eight she announced she wanted to be a schoolteacher, an ambition that she never wavered from and started working steadily towards. Mum and Dad didn't know much about education, they were proud of us just for being happy, well-behaved children and for surviving each year. They weren't interested in pushing us to achieve anything more than they had, maybe because they were perfectly happy as they were and assumed we would be too. They were too busy working, cleaning, cooking, and keeping us fed and warm to look beyond what they had. I remember big Sunday roasts with lots of potatoes and vegetables. We always had butter and never margarine and a nice warm meal every evening of the week. We could often smell Mum's home-baked bread from the end of the road — every time I pass a bakery counter in a supermarket I am reminded of her. Our parents always provided well for us, and we always felt secure and looked after. But they didn't even know Pat was sitting the eleven-plus exam until she came home afterwards and told them.

Pat passed the exam, which meant she could go

to high school. To me, my big sister seemed very special and grown-up. Teachers seemed to come from a different world to the one I knew. My world centred around our estate, but teachers came from somewhere else, where I knew things were done differently, although I didn't quite know how. It seemed so impressive to think Patricia would be becoming one of them, someone that other people looked up to.

Sheila, my second sister who was three years older than me, was the complete opposite; she couldn't even spell. She was sent to be tested at a special school to see if she needed extra help but passed the test, which meant she could stay in the main-stream school.

I was well-behaved at school, always had good reports and always studied hard. I loved it there and at home. By the time I came along, life for my parents was a bit easier, so as the youngest of the family I sometimes felt I was spoiled a little more than the others, and of course I never seemed to mind too much.

One day Mum saw Dad slipping me some money. 'That's his last half-crown he's given you,' she said, perhaps hoping I would take pity on him and give it back.

'I don't care,' I replied, my nose in the air. 'He said I can have it, so it's mine.'

In my defence, my conscience must have been beginning to prick, even at that stage; otherwise I wouldn't remember the incident so clearly all these years later, would I? But that one small memory helps me to understand who I am and the family I have come from, something I have since learned the true value of.

I enjoyed school, but I wasn't really interested in my studies in the way that Pat was, although I didn't have any of the excuses Sheila had. I could have done better if I'd really wanted to, but there were other distractions. I had discovered something that was to become a great passion of mine: dancing. It was all I wanted to do all day. The half-crown from Dad was for a dancing class, which was probably why I couldn't bear to give it back. I had loved dancing for as long as I could remember. When I was four years old, Dad took me to see a Betty Grable film and I was so excited by it that I got up and danced in the aisle. Dad said, 'Sit down, Mavis!'

but the usherettes thought I was sweet and said, 'Oh, go on, let her.' From then on, I danced like mad. But I never wanted to be a ballerina. I loved the dancing in the Hollywood musicals, particularly tap, so I went to all the classes I could.

As the youngest, I was certainly very indulged by my parents and my older sisters. I can remember standing on the kitchen table, having Mum and Sheila make a dancing dress for me. It was beautiful and they were happy to fuss and take trouble over it until it was perfect. I must say, it was lovely to be the centre of attention like that and I loved being looked after so well.

We had a happy childhood, in my opinion. All Mum and Dad ever did was care for us. They never went out looking for a good time and never thought of themselves. The only thing Dad would spend money on for himself was cigarettes, everything else was for us. We were their life and they were totally selfless in their dedication to us, making sure we had everything they could afford to give us. Even though there was rationing, Mum would still manage to get us Easter eggs each year, heaven knows how she managed it.

They always supported us in everything we wanted to do and by their example they showed me just what good parenting should be about, without ever having to put it into words.

When I was ten years old I met two more friends, Sandra and Hilda, and they became as close to me as Rita. We were now a gang of four, going everywhere together, telling each other everything, inseparable for life, and still together today, only now we live in a new century and very different times.

I played for the school netball and rounders teams and often travelled to away matches at other schools. Most of them were in built-up areas and I was shocked to see that people lived in back-to-back houses with no gardens to play in and outside toilets. It made me realise how lucky I was.

Every August, Sandra, Hilda and I would go with Hilda's parents to Blackpool, where we were free to spend our days on the piers listening to Slim Whitman singing 'Rose Marie'. We visited the Winter Gardens and booked to see all the shows.

Every Christmas we would queue up at each of the three Leeds theatres to get the cheapest seats for the pantomimes. On normal days we would just go for walks or sit around in the local park, which had a lovely lake with a café. Another annual ritual was the bonfire in our back garden every 5 November. Mum and Dad would always provide some fireworks and we would sit around the fire until the last ember had died out, never wanting the evening to end.

Sandra, Hilda and I started going to dance classes together. Rita didn't come with us as she wasn't as keen on dancing as the rest of us. From the age of ten we went to the Dorothy Goddard School of Dancing and we would search out any dances we could find going on in the Middleton area, down at the YWCA, at clubs and in the local hall. We seldom strayed out of our area, not even going into Leeds very often, but we still managed to find classes in tap, ballet, modern, anything that was on offer. If there was music, even an out-of-tune piano, and movement, then I was happy. Three times a week we would go to the Tivoli, our local cinema, to watch the likes of Doris Day or Debbie Reynolds star in their latest movie. We would learn the songs and dance routines by heart so we could go home and practise them over and over. I had endless supplies of joy and energy.

Once Pat went away to college there was one less mouth to feed and I could be even more indulged; everything I wanted I got and I wasn't nearly as grateful at the time as I should have been. Looking back, with the help of everything I have learned between then and now, I realise just how fortunate I was. All that is possible because I can remember who I was and what I did in those early years.

2

Keith

I became aware of Keith Marsh's existence on the estate when I was fifteen but I never bothered with him. He went around with a group who were generally thought of as a rough crowd, and he dressed himself up as a Teddy boy with drainpipe trousers and a drape coat. That group thought they were something special, but they didn't impress us. I doubt they actually got up to anything that bad by today's standards, not much more than a bit of swearing and bad manners probably, but they gave off a dangerous air and that was quite enough for four proper young girls like us to make sure our paths didn't cross.

Keith was a bit of a dandy, putting a great deal of thought into his appearance, very unlike my dad and his friends, who were the sort of men I was used to. He even went and got his hair permed once so he would look more like Tony Curtis, who was the big film star and heart-throb of the time. Curtis had a big black quiff of hair and his picture used to be in the window of virtually every barber's shop in the area. It was the 1950s, Elvis Presley was only just starting out on his career and the Beatles were hardly out of school. No one was used to seeing boys preening themselves and dressing like that. Keith and his friends went out with a lot of girls but Rita, Sandra, Hilda and I thought we were above all that. We were four well-behaved but fun-loving girls who enjoyed spending time with boys but were having too good a time to settle down with just one.

The boys used to treat us differently as well, and even stopped swearing when we were around, as if we were young ladies whose sensibilities had to be protected. Or maybe they just knew we were all quite happy to tell them what we thought of them if they pushed their luck. Girls don't always realise just how scared of them boys are at that age, and we were probably more scary than most. But I was actually a gentle child, always keen to avoid confrontations and always tactful with people. I prided myself on speaking my mind nicely.

My friends and I were always top of our classes, but we weren't offered any opportunities for further education; we were simply expected to leave school and go to work at fifteen. We had no particular ambition or goals in life, beyond being able to earn our livings and lead pleasant lives. My sister Pat's example had had no effect on me, and I was quite happy to leave the ambitious, career-minded side of things to her. We weren't rebels and we did the work that was set for us and behaved for the teachers, but we left school as soon as we were old enough, eager to get out of our regimented, narrow existence, earn a bit of money and spend as much time as possible dancing. So at fifteen I went out into the big wide world, full of excitement about being a grown-up at last. Fifteen seems such a young age now, but then, we felt as though we'd done our time at school, got our educations and could finally start living.

My first job was in Dixon's dress shop in the Briggate area of Leeds, where they used to dress up the dummies in the windows to look like different film stars in an attempt to lure the customers in with a bit of Hollywood glamour. I would have to put the labels on them, pointing out to window browsers that the looks they were admiring actually belonged to stars like Betty Grable, Rita Hayworth, Bette Davis or Marilyn Monroe.

Sandra and Hilda were working as shop girls too, Sandra at W.H. Smith and Hilda in a shoe shop. When they got their lunch breaks they would hurry to Dixon's to fetch me and we would go running down to the local Mecca, where Jimmy Savile was starting his career as a disc jockey, playing the early pop and rock'n'roll records, most of which were still coming over from America at that time with stars like Bill Haley and Jerry Lee Lewis. English singers like Cliff Richard and Adam Faith were also bursting on to the scene. It all sounded so new and exciting and full of life, like nothing our parents had ever listened to, and so good to dance to.

We would pay sixpence each to bop together through our lunch hours, before running back to work for the afternoon, invigorated rather than exhausted. We were having a lovely time. I can still recall so many memories from that time, not just the clothes and the music, but the smells as well, like the aroma of fresh roasting coffee that used to assail us when we walked past the doors of Kardomah Café in Briggate. We couldn't actually afford to go in but I used to long to try coffee for myself. I eventually started drinking it when I was twenty-two and I have never lost the taste. Because I'm always on a diet, I drink it black and without sugar.

Jimmy Savile already had a reputation in the area and these were the days when Radio Luxembourg was the only 'pirate' radio station and opportunities were limited for young people to listen to the sort of music they really liked. At the time Jimmy seemed very eccentric and different.

It's hard to remember that such innocent times ever existed, when kids can now hear their music in every shop they walk into, on dozens of different radio and television stations twenty-four hours a day, not to mention from their iPods and car stereos. Now there are thousands of disc jockeys and thousands of clubs, but then it was almost unknown. It was the very beginning of the youth culture that would change everything. We were only dipping our toes in but it would eventually allow our children to have experiences and gain knowledge that we would never even have dreamed existed. Characters like Jimmy Savile were like nothing that had gone before and the whole world was about to change, but we didn't know or care about that, as long as we were allowed to dance.

The four of us saved up so that we could go to Muriel Smith's every week. It was the posh ladies' hairdresser's in town and we would come out with our hair in the latest fashion of high bouffant hairdos, backcombed like mad under the smooth surface and hairsprayed into place. Once, Jimmy was in there too, having his hair bleached, which was an outrageous thing for a man to do in those days, especially so blatantly. We were shocked but secretly very excited to have spotted him.

After about six months the manageress at Dixon's asked me to help out in the cashiers' office and from that moment I was hooked. I loved office work, which was funny because I left school vowing that I never wanted to do anything like schoolwork ever again. But as soon as I started, I realised how much I liked using my brain and working out all the percentages and figures. It turned out I had a very orderly mind and kept it all neat and clear, which helped me to organise things well. Even today I am the same and can put my hand immediately on anything I want in the house. It was obvious that I was much better at working on the accounts than I was at selling the clothes, so that's where I stayed, working out the staff commissions on every item sold. They would get threepence for a coat or dress sold, but they got sixpence in the pound on a wedding dress. They would end up earning more on commission than in their weekly wages. It was a good place to work and the manageress also used to let us put clothes and shoes to one side and pay so much a week for them.

———————

'You've not seen a picture till you've seen *Gone with the Wind*,' Mum always said. It was one of her great favourites but I had never seen it, so when I saw it was ending its run at the Tivoli, I decided to go. It was a Friday night in 1957 and I was seventeen years old.

Hilda, Sandra, Rita and I always went everywhere as a group but on this particular night, they were all busy with their boyfriends. I had had some boyfriends by then, three of them, strangely all called Alan, but I didn't have anyone around that night. Two of those Alans are dead now and the third one has become very rich as a blacksmith and still jokes that he had a narrow escape when I dropped him.

'It doesn't matter,' I said to myself. 'I'll just go on my own.'

It was the first time I'd ever gone to the cinema alone, without either a boyfriend or my gang of girlfriends, but I didn't want to miss the film, so off I went.

When I got to the window to buy my ticket, I bumped into Keith Marsh, who was on his own as well. He was an apprentice working on the railways by then, out of school like me and earning a living, although not a very good one. He was always a real gentleman in his behaviour towards me, even though the boys he ran around with were a bit flirty, so when he suggested we sat together I had no objection.

I'd always thought that Keith was quite good-looking — people later used to say he looked a bit like Paul McCartney, although I don't think anyone would have known who Paul McCartney was at that time — but I was more interested in watching the film, which I enjoyed immensely. It was just as good as Mum had promised, and we sat there in the dark, enthralled by the passionate Scarlet O'Hara and the dashing Rhett Butler.

When we came out into the fresh air, Keith offered to walk me home, which was good of him. After all, he didn't have to. He could easily have just waved me goodbye at the cinema, since we weren't officially on a date.

'Are you doing anything tomorrow evening?' he asked as we strolled back down the avenue.

'I've not got anything planned,' I said.

'Nor have I. I'll meet you, shall I?'

'All right,' I agreed. I tried to make it sound casual, like it wasn't a real date, but the next day I went round to my friend Sandra's house.

'I've agreed to go out with Keith Marsh tonight,' I told her.

'I'll tell you what we'll do,' she suggested. 'Barrie and me will be on the same bus as you, and then we can go out as a foursome.'

Barrie was her boyfriend at the time, and they are still happily married today.

The trams used to run through Middleton in those days, but there were buses as well and Keith and I had arranged to be on the number 29 bus at half past seven. I felt quite excited at the prospect of seeing him again, and more confident now I knew Sandra and Barrie were going to be there too. The plan worked perfectly and we 'accidentally' bumped into one another as soon as we got on the bus. Keith seemed quite happy when we suggested teaming up as a foursome and spending the evening on a pub crawl round Briggate. I was soon to find out that Keith was always very easygoing and seldom turned down an opportunity to spend a few hours in the pub. As we were now officially on a date, and since Sandra and Barrie were there to protect my honour, I allowed him to kiss me a few times and it turned out to be a lovely night. I realised I felt differently about him to any of the other boys I'd been out with and it gradually dawned on me that I was falling for him.

When he suggested we meet again the next night, Sunday, I didn't have any hesitation in agreeing, and didn't feel the need to take chaperones this time. We went back to the cinema again to watch something called *How to Murder a Rich Uncle*, a comedy thriller that had just come out. Sitting together in the double seats, Keith and I missed half of what was going on on-screen, being too absorbed in one another. I don't think they have double seats in cinemas any more, but of course courting couples have more places to meet than they did in our day. You couldn't take a boyfriend or girlfriend home and expect any privacy, so a darkened cinema was our best chance of having somewhere comfortable, warm and private for a bit of a kiss and cuddle. I was beginning to realise just what a good man he was, and I would still be discovering new depths and strengths to his character forty years later.

From that first weekend together, we started going out on a regular basis but it was about six months before I realised that I had fallen in love and that he was the one for me. After that there was never another man for me and, I hope, never another girl for Keith. We saw each other virtually every night. My family didn't seem to mind Keith, though they didn't see much of him really. When he came round, he'd knock on the door and then I'd come rushing out and we'd go off together. I went round to his house though, to meet his parents. His older sisters were both married and had left home, so it was only Keith living there, and we all got on very well and liked each other a lot.

When he turned eighteen, Keith decided he was never going to earn enough working for the railways and went for a job down the pits instead, pushing coal around. It was a hard life, but there weren't many choices for the boys from round our area in those days. Even then, Keith was never frightened of a bit of hard work.

We'd been together for over two years and it seemed like the natural thing when we decided to get married. By then I was just two months off being twenty and he was a year older. There was nothing unusual in getting married so young in those days; in fact, it was what was expected. Many girls had started having babies by that time. Nowadays, everyone makes such careful financial plans about their futures together, putting off having kids until just the right moment, but then everyone did the same as everyone else and no one gave it a lot of thought: you left school, met a boy, got married and had a family.

Keith took money very seriously, which was another reason I admired him. He was earning about £3 10s a week (which wasn't much even in those days before inflation), but he had already managed to save about £7, which was a lot of money then, when most young men were spending their wages almost the moment they were given them. Not only was he handsome, it seemed he was going to be the sort to look after a girl as well. Discovering all this about him was a revelation to me. It just went to show that you can't jump to conclusions about someone just because of the way they look and the company they keep. I had learned a valuable lesson, not to be so quick to judge in future.

I might have been on the verge of becoming a married woman, but as far as my family were concerned, I was still behaving like the spoiled little sister I had always been. When we started to lay plans for the wedding I insisted I wanted my reception held at Betty's Café in Leeds, which seemed really posh to me. While everyone else we knew had a corned-beef tea or boiled-egg sandwiches at their receptions, I wanted a proper sit-down roast dinner, unheard of for council-house people in those days, but eventually I got my way. It cost my poor dad twelve and six a head, but he never complained. It was very expensive – Keith's total savings would only have paid for eleven people and we had thirty guests, and a bus to take everyone from Middleton to Leeds. The bus was from Watsons, a bus company near our house – I used to babysit for the owners so I knew them well.

Although I had been christened a Catholic, I had never gone to church as a child or to a Catholic school, which meant I had to go to the priest for some lessons so I could be confirmed before the wedding ceremony. When the priest heard I was planning to marry the notorious Keith Marsh, he was horrified. It seemed I wasn't the only one who judged by appearances, although a priest of all people ought to have looked a little deeper before jumping to conclusions.

'You're not going to marry him, are you?' he asked, not bothering for a second to hide his feelings.

Keith was also a Catholic and at the time his mother used to send him off to church every now and then. It seemed he had been going to confession and this priest knew all about his past track record with girlfriends. Even then it seemed very wrong for a priest to express any opinion at all when he hadn't been asked. It wasn't as if I was planning to have an affair with a married man, or was getting married because I had to. But those were the days when authority figures like priests could do more or less as they liked and everyone rushed around trying to impress them, saying 'yes sir, no sir'. Although it was the beginning of the sixties and more and more young people were starting to question all forms of authority such as priests, doctors, teachers and politicians, this had not quite reached our quiet housing estate outside Leeds.

By that stage, however, nothing would have put me off marrying Keith. I just listened to what the priest had to say, kept quiet and got on with laying my plans for the big day just the same. By then I was completely confident that I knew Keith better than the priest did, even if I had never been privileged to hear Keith's confession. I had decided this was the man I was going to marry, just as I had decided I was going to have my reception at Betty's Café; it would take more than a bit of disapproval from a priest to change my mind. Neither of my parents, whose opinions I did respect, had any problem with my choice at all and finally the big day arrived and our wedding went like a dream.

My poor sister Pat, who had worked so hard to get her qualifications and become a teacher, had to pay for her own wedding that year because my parents had spent all their money on mine. I excused myself with the thought that she was earning more than I was as an office girl but, thinking back, I'm amazed she wasn't more resentful than she was. I always seemed to get away with these things.

Within a few months of our getting married, Sandra had married Barrie, Rita had married Arthur and Hilda had married Bill. So all eight of us went to Blackpool together for a joint honeymoon. We danced the week away, young, in love and in the first year of the 'Swinging Sixties'. We had a marvellous time before we returned back to Middleton to settle down to our new married lives and the big adventure that awaited us.

Keith's parents were just as lovely as mine, and his father was an angel, doing everything for his family, just like my dad. Looking at him, and seeing so much of him in Keith, I knew I had chosen a good man. His dad worked as an engineer and boiler man at R.W. Crabtree, which later became Crabtree Vickers, a big local employer.

There is so much written today about how hard it is for young people 'to get a foot on the housing ladder' because property is so expensive, but it was always so, particularly in those days when nobody wanted to give mortgages to anyone who didn't already have money in the bank, and when it was virtually impossible to build up enough savings for a deposit. Most young couples had to start off their married lives by staying with one or other of their families, or living in a rented room till they could afford to buy or rent a home of their own, or reached the top of a council-housing waiting list. Keith was the youngest of three children, just like me, and as both of his sisters were married – one, Colleen, had emigrated to Canada – there was some spare room at his parents' house and we moved in there for the first year of our married life while we saved up as much as possible for a home of our own.

Dad liked to talk to everyone in the neighbourhood as he went on his bin rounds, and always knew exactly what was going on. He heard about a one-up, one-down house for sale not far away for £250. It was a lot of money, considerably more than a whole year of Keith's wages working down the coal pits, but it seemed worth trying to get a mortgage to cover it. We went to see the man who owned it and he must have taken pity on us because he told us not to bother about getting a mortgage, just to give him ten pounds a month till it was all paid off. We were very grateful, knowing just how tough building societies could be to young would-be buyers.

Both of us were meticulous about paying our debts on time. My dad had always drummed it into me that the one thing you should always make sure you've got is a roof over your head. 'Whatever you do,' he would say, 'pay for your rent first.'

We could see what he meant. People round our way were often being forced to do 'moonlight flits' because they weren't able to make the rent payments; they'd let their debts build up, and now they knew the bailiffs were on their way. We used to watch them doing it late at night, after we got home from the pictures or dancing, as they loaded up vans with all their possessions and disappeared into the darkness in search of somewhere new to settle until their debts caught up with them again. It was a never-ending cycle for people like that and neither Keith nor I ever wanted to be in that position. We wanted to be able to sleep soundly in our beds at night like our parents, not fearing every knock on the door and every letter through the letter box.

Our first proper home was like one of the houses I had been so horrified by when I was a child, but to us now it seemed like a tiny doll's house. It had a front door opening straight on to the road and a toilet out the back, but it seemed wonderful to us. I was working as a telephonist at the GPO by then (which was the company that was later split up to become the Post Office and British Telecom), and Keith left the pits to take a job with his dad at Crabtree Boilers as a boiler man; nowadays he'd be known as something much more impressive, like a heating engineer, but then he was perfectly happy to be a boiler man. I was glad that he was out of the mines and in the fresh air, but he was still having to work incredibly hard. At that stage he was working sixty hours a week to make enough money to get us started in life, because the only way people like us could hope to get off the council estates was by working longer hours than anyone else. Those were the days when the workers were still expected to take their caps off to management, but Keith wouldn't have worn one anyway in case it spoiled his hair. He was the best husband and provider any girl could have asked for, I was so proud of him.

We were a very happy, young married couple, with a group of good friends, our health and our jobs. Life and the future were bright for us.

3

Starting a Family

Although our little doll's house was perfect for the two of us, we were ready to move on three years later, when I fell pregnant for the first time. Deciding to sell it and use the money as a deposit on a more suitable family home, we found a man who was willing to pay us £280, which seemed like a good profit to us. Nobody expected to make money from their homes in the sixties. It wasn't until the seventies that property prices started to rise so steeply and homeowners suddenly found themselves far richer than they had ever planned.

Until then house prices had always stayed pretty stable, just like the value of the pound in your pocket.

The deal to sell our little house seemed all set to go through when the buyer came round to see us unexpectedly. His face was grim as he told us that he had been to the council's offices to check the deeds of the house and had discovered that it was in a 'grey area'.

'What's a grey area?' we asked.

He told us that it meant the house was going to be compulsorily purchased by the council for demolition, to make way for a new housing scheme. It was the first we'd heard of it, but it meant we couldn't sell it to anyone else because they would know it was going to be demolished, even though we hadn't been told. In the end, the council paid us only about forty pounds for the property we had been pinning all our hopes on, which was a big disappointment, but at least it gave us some money to use as a deposit on our next home.

It was a shock to us, because we had always been told by the people whose opinions we respected that the safest place to put your money was into bricks and mortar. It was an unsettling reminder that nothing is ever certain, that you can lay your plans as carefully as you like, but there can still be the unexpected event that will make a mockery of the whole idea that we have control over our own destinies. It was a lesson we would soon forget, and would have to be reminded of with terrible suddenness nearly thirty years later.

These little setbacks always seem like the end of the world at the time, but now that I look back, losing money on that house sale wasn't so bad. We were still only in our early twenties and hardly anyone that we knew of our age had even bought their first house by then. We were all struggling together, but we were still managing to keep our heads above water. It just seemed unfair that the council were able to take our home from us, without proper recompense, and that we were so helpless to do anything about it.

Life went on though, and we managed to move anyway. Our next home was on a nice new estate, which has become a no-go area in recent years because of violence and crime, but then it was lovely. The house had underfloor heating, three bedrooms and a big garden. We thought we were in heaven when we moved in and were able to spread ourselves out a bit. Indoor plumbing was also a relief with a baby on the way.

I gave birth to my first daughter when I was twenty-four, which was older than most of the girls around the estate but it still felt like a frightening venture into the unknown to us. I didn't even have any idea what to call her, so Patricia, my teacher sister, went through all the names of the children in her class at school. One of them was called Gaynel, which I thought sounded really pretty and unusual. Patricia asked the girl what it meant and she said it was the name of a Welsh songbird, and it turned out her mother was called Mavis too; so it seemed like fate was trying to give us a clue, and we called our little girl Gaynel Ruth. I gave her a plain second name so that she could use that if she didn't like the fancy one.

I had left the GPO by then and had gone to work for British Gas as a clerk. Because we had a mortgage and planned to give our children as good a lifestyle as possible, I didn't want to give up work, and luckily for us my parents were more than happy to help us in any way they could. They looked after Gaynel for me while I was at work. Dad had retired from the bins by then and wanted something to concentrate his energies on now that all his own children had grown up and gone off into the world. He took his childcare duties with his new granddaughter just as seriously as he had with my sisters and me. He used to take Gaynel out in her pushchair on five-mile walks every day. When she started walking for herself at eighteen months, she immediately demanded to go out on foot with him, leaving the pushchair behind, and as her legs grew stronger the two of them would cover miles together, talking all the time. I liked having an office job and came home in the evenings keen to spend time with my baby, which I might not have done if I had been looking after her all day. It was a brilliant arrangement.

I think one of the greatest gifts that any adult can give to a child is to spend time talking to them as an equal, rather than patronising them. We're all in such a hurry the whole time that it is sometimes hard to find the time to slow down and just answer their questions properly, especially when they're little and their questions seem so daft and repetitive most of the time. I'm sure Gaynel was born with a high intelligence, but I am also sure that the stimulation she received from having so much of my father's undivided attention in those early years helped to mould her into the adult she was to become. By the time she went to school at four she could already read and could recognise virtually every animal in the world.

Gaynel's progress seemed normal to me and it wasn't until I started to mix with other young mums at her first school that I realised just how bright and far ahead she was. But her intelligence was only one of her strengths. Sometimes a clever child can be hard to bring up because they're always challenging their parents or becoming bored, but Gaynel seemed to be a perfect child in every way. She never answered us back, was never naughty, and always did whatever I asked of her without complaining.

If I tell her now how good she was as a child, she claims I frightened her into obedience when she was tiny by telling her I would give her to the gypsies if she didn't behave and she would 'finish up with jam in her hair'. I can't imagine why I would have said such a thing, but she is certain I did and it obviously made a big impact on her. I do remember that when she got older I would threaten her with boarding school if she misbehaved, even though there wasn't a chance we would ever be able to afford such a luxury, or would have considered it even if we could. But they were obviously very effective threats because I have no memory of her ever playing me up.

Despite her claim that her mother put the fear of God into her, Gaynel always seemed like a really happy child, passing her eleven-plus when she was only nine and going on to Notre Dame High School when she was ten. Every morning she and her friend, Teresa, would catch a bus all the way across Leeds to be taught by the nuns.

Although I wasn't devout myself, I wanted the children brought up Catholic. I felt it was the best way to provide a foundation in a religion for them so that they could choose what they wanted to do later in life. They were all christened as babies, and later confirmed into the Church. As it happened, it also meant that the children had very good educations, because the local Catholic schools were excellent, with high academic standards and good discipline. It gave all the children a wonderful start in life, so that they could make the most of their natural talents, and I'm very grateful for that.

Gaynel was such a lovely child that I hadn't really felt the need to have any more. I thought that life would be so easy with one perfect child, and we would be able to indulge her far more than if we had other mouths to feed. But although I hadn't planned to, I fell pregnant a couple of years after she was born and in 1967 our second daughter, Dena Rebecca, came along.

Dena was very different to her sister, always comical and never serious. When she was three she developed a terrible limp. I took her to the doctor and he referred her to a specialist, who couldn't find anything wrong. It turned out that all she was doing was copying a neighbour who had a bad leg. She kept the performance up for six months before deciding she'd had enough of limping and cheerfully confessed. She always said she wanted to be an actress and it wasn't hard to imagine her doing it.

We were very happy with our two little daughters, and we felt like a real family.

Now that he'd got a taste of being a homeowner, Keith soon started wanting to move on and found a bungalow just up the road from where we were. It was in a terrible state inside, but it was still a lovely house even though it only had two bedrooms and the place we were in had three. Nevertheless, it was so nice and we didn't see why we needed a lot of bedrooms with only two daughters so we bought it for £3,950 and moved in in 1969. Keith went to work as normal on the day of the move and my mum and I had us all moved in, unpacked, the beds made, everything washed and ironed and tea ready by the time he came home in the evening. Life just seemed to be very simple and very manageable. Nothing cropped up that I didn't feel I could control and cope with. I was extremely happy with my life. I had two beautiful children, a lovely husband and a new home, which I was sure we could make as nice as the last one had been.

Despite the misgivings of the priest who had warned me off marrying him, Keith was proving to be a super husband and father, although he did still like his beer now and then. Every Friday night he would go to the club for a few drinks, but otherwise he came home every evening. I could have gone to the pub with him if I'd asked Mum to have the girls for me, but she had usually had them all day and it didn't seem fair to ask. I certainly didn't begrudge Keith his one night out a week when he worked as hard as he did.

I never lost my taste for dancing during those years and we would often go out as a foursome on Saturday nights, with Sandra and me on the dance floor and Barrie and Keith watching us, grinning from the bar, happy to let us have our few hours in the spotlight, letting off steam just as we had ever since we were fifteen.

One of the great advantages of the bungalow was that it backed on to the indoor swimming pool of the local school. The public were allowed to use it once the kids had gone home, but hardly anyone did; usually it was just us, and sometimes the headmaster and his family. I used to take the girls over whenever I could because I thought it was important that children learned to swim as soon as possible, for safety reasons as well as because it was good exercise. We were so close I didn't even have to dry myself off when I got out of the water. I would just run quickly across the garden with the girls to get changed in the comfort of our own home.

Everything in our lives seemed so perfect and under control that once again we didn't think we would risk having any more children. Two little girls seemed the perfect amount. So at the end of the year Keith booked himself in for a vasectomy in the following February. But at Christmas I discovered I was already pregnant again. When we found out, we laughed — after all that careful planning, we were going to have another baby after all. I was sure it was going to be another girl and I was very happy because I loved Gaynel and Dena, and I knew they'd enjoy having a baby sister to play with. So we planned to call her Keely Rachel.

The following August I gave birth to my third

and last child, Keith having safely had his vasectomy by that time. But when Keely Rachel arrived, she turned out to be a boy, and we called him Matthew Clayton.

It was lovely to have a son and Matthew soon turned out to be just as good and easy to bring up as his sisters. Dena, who was about three when he arrived, was obsessed with her little baby brother, wanting to look after him all the time, like he was a real live doll.

Right from the start, I never had to worry about Matthew. He was an angelic baby and, as he grew up, a calm, sensible child everyone loved. He was always well-behaved and obedient. Because we lived on the main road, for instance, all the children had strict instructions never to go out of the gate on their own. Even when Matthew was seven, he would still come in to ask me if it was all right for him for go out and retrieve a football that had escaped over the wall. He was the most easy-going child imaginable. I decided at that stage he was old enough and sensible enough to be allowed in and out of the gate without permission. When I told him he simply thanked me politely. He never questioned the rules I laid down, or tried to push the boundaries.

I had some quite strict rules, like never dropping litter or going on to other people's property. I was pretty firm by nature and liked to have my life neat and under control, but none of the kids ever seriously rebelled against my instructions or made things difficult for me. When I saw the way that some other people's children behaved, I counted myself very lucky. At the time I think I believed their good behaviour was due to the firm way we were bringing them up, but I have seen enough badly-behaved children now to know that sometimes it doesn't matter what the parents do, they just can't control them. In fact, it can often seem that the stricter the parents are, the more the children rebel and cause trouble. I'm not saying that my kids didn't ever stand up to me, because none of them have weak characters, they just always did it with reasoned arguments and persuasion. Dena, in particular, used to argue with me sometimes, but always straight to my face, never going behind my back. It was always over trivial things; for instance, she wasn't one for going to bed if she wasn't tired, even if I told her to, whereas Gaynel was always wanting to go to sleep. Gaynel would never answer me back, but Dena later told me that sometimes, once she was out of my earshot, Gaynel would let rip about what she thought of my maternal firmness.

I have a bit of a reputation for being outspoken, a bit bossy even. I know it's how I come across, and I sometimes wish I didn't, but there's nothing I can do to change my nature, or my strong Yorkshire accent. I know it doesn't always make me seem very nice to people when they first meet me, but it's the way I am and most people are able to see past the loud talk pretty quickly once they get to know me. I speak my mind but there's also another side to me: I'm honest and loyal to my friends. So you take the rough with the smooth with me.

I wanted our children to have happy childhoods, full of lovely memories to treasure when they grew up. When Matthew was almost five, we were walking past a pet shop in town together and saw some collie-cross puppies in the window, crawling all over one another, panting in the heat.

I've never liked dogs much, or any animals for that matter, but I could see Matthew was entranced and I thought he deserved a treat. They were charging £4 for the puppies and I could see that Matthew really wanted one, so I weakened. Of course, as is always the way with these things, it wasn't so much the puppy that cost the money, it was all the accessories it needed, like the basket and the collar and the food. I was very nervous that I had taken on something I was not going to be able to control.

When we got home with our new puppy, Gaynel, who was eleven by then, was furious.

'We can't afford a dog,' she protested, sounding more like she was my mother than my daughter.

'Family allowance will pay for it,' I said, trying to justify my unusually spontaneous extravagance to myself as much as to her.

'You're not having my family allowance for that dog,' she stormed.

But Benjy, as we christened him, soon won her over just like the rest of us. He was the most lovely, obedient of dogs, always desperate to please and we all loved him immensely.

They say that you don't know how happy you are until it's gone, and I think that's true. Life for our family was so easy and happy, and we seemed to have a never-ending supply of luck. We never ran into the kind of problems that plagued other families we knew. Our home was secure and comfortable, our children well-behaved, intelligent and a pleasure to be with – even our dog was loved by everyone. I didn't mean to get complacent, and often tried to count my blessings, but I'm afraid I was so used to things going well that I rather took it for granted. It never occurred to me that our luck might change and our good fortune come to an end. I felt so in charge of my life that I couldn't imagine how it could all be transformed in a moment and hurtle out of my control. I was so sure of myself and my own abilities to cope with anything that fate might throw up, I couldn't imagine things going wrong.

But you never know what is waiting for you round the corner. And I'm glad I didn't know what was coming, because I enjoyed those years with my children to the full, thinking that our golden life would go on for ever, without a cloud to mar it.

I certainly never expected our happiness to end so abruptly.

4

Open All Hours

In 1981, when Matthew was eleven, Keith and I decided to go into business for ourselves. It's a big jump when you have always worked for a regular wage to decide to go out on your own. I had always been particularly cautious in my choice of job, always going for big, blue-chip employers like the GPO, British Gas and Leeds Council, knowing that these companies offered better prospects and equal pay for their female employees. But, just as we had taken the plunge when we decided to become homeowners and then to start a family, now we felt it was the time to be brave and try something new, something we could work on and build up together.

Keith gave up his job as a boiler man and I gave up working at Leeds City Council as a clerk in the cleansing department, and we bought a little local shop, selling everything from baked beans to newspapers. In 1987, we saw another shop a few streets away for sale at a good price and thought we should expand while we could so we bought that as well. Both shops were within walking distance of our house.

If we had realised how much work it would take to run those shops, I don't know that we would ever have plucked up the courage to do it. The one we worked in ourselves most of the time was a bit like the shop depicted in the television series *Open All Hours* with Ronnie Barker and David Jason. We would have to get in at six in the morning to sort out the newspapers and get ready for opening, and we were often still there in the evening, stocktaking and serving customers who had just remembered they didn't have anything for tea. In between, there would be trips to the cash and carry, dealing with tenants and employees, shelf stacking and everything else that makes a shop into the place we all take for granted as customers.

Our bank manager was very understanding about backing us and the business made us a good living in the early days, but it took up almost every waking moment of our lives. I had always enjoyed office life for its social side and for the fact that I could pack up at the end of the working day and not give the job another thought until I arrived back again the following day. It was never like that with the shops, and we both grew more and more exhausted, until eventually we started to make silly mistakes. We used to have a bacon slicer and one evening I sliced the tip of my finger off. Incredibly, I still managed to keep serving the customer so they didn't realise anything was wrong.

I hated working in the shops from the first day, but we had invested all our money into them and so we were committed to making a go of it.

All three children continued to behave immaculately, although Dena was never as straightforward as her older sister had been. She had followed Gaynel to Notre Dame High School, but she didn't like it. Gaynel had been very happy to accept the discipline that the nuns handed out, but Dena was always questioning everything she was told to do. Gaynel loved wearing a school uniform, for instance, whereas Dena hated it, and she didn't like the idea of being in a single-sex school either. She made it clear she was going to leave as soon as she was allowed to. She also encouraged Matthew to stand up for himself as well. When he passed the exam to go to Leeds Grammar at thirteen, we thought he would be pleased. He was always so easygoing, just letting the current of life wash him along, and we assumed this move would be no different.

'I don't want to go,' he announced to Dena.

'Then don't go,' she advised in her usual no-nonsense style.

'Mum,' he said a little later, having thought over his sister's straight-talking advice, 'I don't want to go to Leeds Grammar.'

'You're going to Leeds Grammar,' I said in my usual no-argument voice, shocked that he had finally answered back but expecting him to shrug and give up arguing the moment I put my foot down.

'I'm not,' he insisted calmly. 'I don't want to go.'

When he started to explain himself I could see the sense of his thinking. That's how it always seemed to work with me. I would say the first thing that came into my head with huge certainty, but would always be willing to change my mind once someone who might have put a little more thought into the subject put their case forward. Matthew believed that if he went to a school like that he would start to speak differently, and then he would no longer fit in around Middleton. For instance, at the grammar school they referred to the dining hall, rather than the canteen. In fact, we only ever went back into the estates when we went to visit my mum, who still lived in the house where I had been brought up, so I doubt if he would have lost many friends, but I understood the principle of what he was saying. As he was so adamant and we didn't want to make him do something he was uncomfortable with, we started looking for an alternative.

We decided our best option would be another Catholic school, as the girls had responded so well to theirs — if you didn't count Dena finding the regime a bit stricter than she would have liked — and we found that Mount St Mary's, which had previously been all girls, had just started taking boys. It was a good school and they agreed to accept Matthew. We wanted him to go somewhere that would stretch his imagination and catch his interest. We could tell that Matthew, like his sisters, was bright and would get further in the world than us if he had the right education.

Matthew's childhood seemed to be a happy one. He was always well and never seemed to have accidents, except when he broke a finger once at school playing with a medicine ball. He wasn't the reckless type, although he enjoyed riding about on his bike more than we realised at the time. When Keith and I were working in the shop, we'd tell him to stay around near us and not to go too far. Then, when he was about fourteen, we went to Rothwell, which is a few miles away from our shops, and he said casually, 'I used to cycle around here.' We were both very surprised, at which point it came out that Matthew wasn't quite the obedient boy we'd thought and wasn't averse to heading off on his own little adventures when he felt like it. Perhaps that's more healthy than being a complete little angel.

He was like any normal boy — he had hobbies and loved the stars and the night sky. He loved climbing, and was always clambering over anything he could find, from his bunk bed to trees in the garden. He wasn't particularly into sport, and neither is Keith, so we didn't have one of those football-obsessed households. He and Keith were as close as they could be, considering that we were working all hours. So when Keith wasn't in the shop, he would teach Matthew gymnastics in the garden. They happily passed hours like this, learning hand springs and attempting somersaults.

Although we'd left school early ourselves, a good education was something we valued highly and wanted for our children. Occasionally, we would be sure that we were right about things to do with our children and wanted to fight our corner, even though we didn't always have the vocabularies with which to wage our battles as diplomatically as perhaps we should have done. Matthew had already told us he wanted to go to university when he left school and I knew that for the physics course he wanted to do he would need to get a maths O level. So when the school told us they were going to move him down to the CSE class, I went in one parents' evening and put my foot down.

My mum and dad would never have done such a thing. Education was never much of an issue in my family or in Keith's, and not really discussed. It wasn't much of a priority among the people who taught us either, to be honest. I remember one of my teachers saying once that all he was turning out at our school was 'factory fodder'. Their only aim was to get their pupils reading and writing, and keep them under control until they were ready to unleash them on to the employment market. You don't need many qualifications for work down a mine or on an assembly line.

But when it came to our children, we wanted more. When the teachers weren't that keen to listen to us about Matthew and his maths, we fell back on plain old-fashioned stubbornness. We simply refused to change our minds and loudly told them exactly what we wanted – we weren't going to give up on Matthew's chances, even if the teachers were. It paid off and Matthew was moved back to the O-level class. And fortunately, he passed the exam without too much trouble, so our obstinacy had been more than worth it.

At eighteen, after her A levels, Gaynel went to Trent Poly to get a degree. She joined a four-year course in accountancy, which included working at Rolls-Royce during the third year. But she lost interest after that and dropped out of the fourth year, saying she didn't want to 'number crunch' for the rest of her life. She did a one-year teacher-training course but decided that wasn't for her either. In her late thirties she went back to college and got a first-class degree in pure maths, proving to everyone, including herself, what a brilliant brain she had. Dena left school at sixteen and went on a photography course. She also went to university later in life and gained a 2.1 degree in art, psychology and history at Leeds University.

Although we wanted all of the children to go on to further education, we weren't worried when Dena left at sixteen because she was so full of plans and self-confidence that we were sure she would achieve whatever she set out to do. As soon as she could, she went off and got a flat of her own so she could live independently and please herself. We never had any worries that she would be all right.

Despite the fact that our parents had never asked anything of us in that way, Keith and I both expected our children to get an education, and they seemed to expect the same. We never pushed them to be ambitious or nagged them to do their home-work, like some parents seemed to have to. Our three just got on with it. We were lucky that, being Catholic, we had access to such good schools that provided a positive learning atmosphere and expected high standards. All my friends' children went to the same schools that Keith and I went to, and none of them went on to do degrees.

Before long, it was only Matthew left at home. Gaynel had already met Bill, whom she would later marry, and had gone to live with him in Birmingham. Dena was off exploring the world, something she has never stopped doing.

Everything had always gone so well for all three of our children that we never had any fears for any of their futures. We were sending them out into the world well equipped to make their livings and look after themselves: educated, respectable citizens who would contribute to society.

But soon, a disaster that no one could possibly have predicted would change everything.

5

Falling in Love

When he was fifteen, Matthew met Ivona, a Polish girl, and fell in love. They were besotted with each other and we were delighted and happy to encourage them in any way we could. We liked Ivona a lot and we could see that it made him very happy to be with her. When Matthew passed his A levels in physics, maths and chemistry, we treated them both to the reward of a holiday together in Majorca, where Gaynel's future father-in-law had an apartment that they could borrow.

Ivona's father was a doctor at Leeds Infirmary and

I'm not sure he was too pleased about his seven-teen-year-old daughter going off on holiday with her boyfriend, especially when the boyfriend was a lad from the Middleton area, but he was kind enough not to try to stop them. They had a fantastic time together and came back tanned, healthy and glowing. They were so obviously happy together, it was hard to imagine them ever apart.

Every year on his birthday Ivona used to bake Matthew wonderful cakes. One year it was in the shape of a blue Cortina, because that was the car he was driving. They used to go and play golf on a course near to her home, and one afternoon another player just gave Matthew a pair of golfing shoes, not wanting anything in return. He was so chuffed when he got home, not able to believe the kindness of a complete stranger.

In 1988, with his A levels under his belt, Matthew took up a place at Sheffield University when he was eighteen to read physics and astronomy. My last baby had flown the nest but I didn't have the time to miss any of them. Keith and I had every hour of the day filled with running the shops and our own lives. The children's independence had grown so gradually and naturally that we had hardly even noticed it. Almost without us realising, they had grown up into independent adults. Their childhoods were over but we had plenty of other things to occupy our thoughts. We saw all three of them regularly and had such good relationships with them that we had no reason to feel sad that they were no longer around all the time. It felt natural that they were off pursuing their own passions and exploring life just as we had.

I think it must always be hard for young couples when they move away to universities and are separated by miles. It's hard enough to keep relationships going in the early stages when you can see each other every day, or at least every weekend. But students don't have the time or the money to come home whenever they want to, or to travel between different universities. I suppose it's easier now that everyone has mobile phones and can call one another on a regular basis, but Matthew and Ivona didn't have that luxury. When you are away from home for the first time, trying to get used to living independently and setting your own work schedules, the last thing you want is to have your mind constantly wandering on to someone you are missing who is living miles away. Part of the attraction about university life is meeting new people, particularly members of the opposite sex, but if you are already in a serious relationship it must be hard to relax while everyone around you is having fun, meeting new people and experimenting with new relationships.

I know Matthew found it hard to be parted from Ivona and every month or so he would come home to see her. On his birthday that first year apart, she baked him a cake in the shape of a telescope, since looking at the stars had now become his obsession. Lots of boys go science- and space-mad when they are young but grow out of it later – Matthew didn't though. His interest just got deeper and deeper and he was determined to learn all he could about the universe, which was reflected in the degree course he chose.

The following year Ivona went to York University and Matthew's worst fears were realised when she met someone else. She finished with him the Christmas of 1989. They had been together for four years by that time, nearly a fifth of his young life, and the break-up devastated him. I think he had assumed they would always be together, as so many young men do when they first fall in love – and maybe I had thought the same. After all, it had worked for Keith and me, and for many of our friends, although we had never been put to the test of spending that much time apart from one another. I imagine it is always harder to keep a relationship going if you spend a great deal of time apart and in the company of unattached people.

Matthew and I didn't talk a lot about personal subjects at that stage, but I could tell that he was grief-stricken. I don't think many young men want to discuss their love lives with their mothers, and most mothers would prefer not to have too many details anyway. After the break-up, though, he did tell me, in his usual quiet, understated way, that he didn't think he would ever love again, not in the way he had loved Ivona. Although it was the sort of melodramatic statement any young lover might make at a moment of heartbreak, I had a feeling it might turn out to be true. She had seemed like the love of his life.

'She's broken my heart,' he admitted, and, as a

mother, I felt my own heart break a little for him. It was so hard to see my son suffering, and to understand how anyone could not love him.

That's not to say that Matthew was on his own for long. He was almost never without a girlfriend. He was very attractive to women, not just because he had lovely dark hair and blue eyes, but also because he was funny and charming and, like his father, a real gentleman. He genuinely liked women – he enjoyed their company and was very caring and considerate towards them. It's no wonder he had no shortage of girlfriends. Men like Matthew are rare and very prized – I know, because he's just like his dad.

But I could see that none of the replacements had got to him in quite the same way Ivona had. They were all nice, pretty girls, but it was never the same. He only ever lasted a year with each one.

In June 1991 Matthew graduated from Sheffield University with a first-class degree in physics and astronomy. Not only did he get a first, he also won something called the Hicks Prize, which was a £200 award for the best student of the year. He told us that he wanted to stay in education and go to Leicester

University to study for a PhD in astrophysics and space science. We were astonished. Our son, it seemed, was turning out to be a bit of a boffin. Not content with all the wonderful things he had seen and done on earth, it seemed he now wanted to explore the entire universe. His world was expanding beyond anything we could have dreamed about. From my dad, who was happy with his local bin round and never wanted to leave the country again after the First World War, we had gone in two generations to a boy who wanted to explore the stars and learn everything there was to know about the heavens. From a family that had barely had any interest in education at all until my sister announced she wanted to be a teacher, we had reached a point where our son wanted to take education as far as he possibly could.

It was something of a golden age in England for people like our children who wanted to go to university because there were no tuition fees and the government was willing to give them grants so they could finance the whole thing without going into debt. And they didn't even have to distract themselves from their studies by getting a job in order to survive. Nowadays students come out with huge debts to pay off, but by the time Matthew eventually finished his PhD, after seven years of higher education, his bank account was still £200 in credit. I dare say not every student was as wise or careful with their money as he was, but many of them were. There was no way we would ever have been able to afford to pay for three children to go to university before grants were available, and I'm very glad that they never had to take on immense loans either. I think the British government of that period should feel proud of what they did for that generation.

When Matthew got his gown for the graduation ceremony at Sheffield he tried to convince me it didn't mean anything to him, but I could see, by the way he and his friends preened themselves in those traditional robes, that they were proud of what they had achieved. Keith and I were certainly proud, and a little amazed, by all three of our lovely, clever children.

'So what do you think you'll do for a career once you've got all these qualifications?' I asked Matthew one day.

'I think,' he replied with only a hint of a smile,

'that I will get myself a basement and make didgeri-
doos.'

It didn't seem that unlikely a picture. He was something of a hippie by that stage, with his long dark hair
knotted into dreadlocks. It was a shock when you
first saw them but they made him look rather glam-
orous and wild. He was never happier than when he
was camping in the mud at Glastonbury, or travelling around the world to different observatories, with
virtually no luggage beyond what he stood up in. In
Germany he gave a lecture, in South Africa he went
up Table Mountain to observe the heavens.

There was never any telling what his next interest
would be. He even joined a juggling club at university, to give himself a break from all the academic
work. The skills needed to keep several balls or clubs
in the air at any one time are very different to the
ones needed to understand some complex problem
of astrophysics, so I suppose that it must have been
a bit like exercising different muscles in his brain,
keeping separate pathways clear, making new
connections and sharpening existing ones.

The month after Matthew graduated in June
1991, Gaynel married Bill in a lovely ceremony in

Manchester, where they were living. It was a wonderful family day that I will always remember, and the following year we welcomed our first grandson, Christian, and then in 1993 our granddaughter Philippa, known as Pippa. We absolutely adored Gaynel's children, who were as charming and sunny-natured as their mother, and we loved being grandparents. It was a very happy time.

Matthew spent four years working on his PhD at Leicester and from what Keith and I could tell he adored every minute of it, although he didn't come home as often, now that he was dating girls down there rather than coming back to see Ivona. He didn't even ring that often now that he was grown up and launched into a life of his own. I remember him calling from Sheffield once while he was still doing his degree. It was the night the Berlin Wall came down in 1989. He was so excited. Watching that wall come down must have been as momentous for his generation as watching Neil Armstrong walking on the moon was for ours.

Usually when he rang he was about to go out to

the pub with his friends and didn't have much time to talk. We didn't mind though, we were just relieved that all three of our children had grown up to be such happy, independent people. We had enough on our minds with the running of the shops and our own social lives not to dwell on what our children might be up to when they were out of our sight. We loved them all dearly, but we were quite content to be getting on with our own lives now that they were grown up.

Matthew started travelling in earnest, going to places that had observatories where he could study the night sky through telescopes. He was a fearless traveller, so different from my father who had never wanted to set foot outside his country again. Matthew would arrive in a strange town or at a foreign airport with nothing more than a compass and would happily walk to wherever he needed to go. Nothing in the world seemed to daunt him, no possibilities seemed to be closed to him. Dena had a similar attitude in many ways, never staying in one job more than about six months, always training to give herself new skills and to open doors both in her mind and her career. They seemed to have none of the caution or inhibition that our generation had been burdened with. Keith and I had been lucky to escape without being turned into 'factory fodder' as that teacher had put it, but our children had total freedom to be or do whatever they chose in life.

In 1989 we sold the first shop and in 1993 Keith and I finally decided that even one was too much work and we set about converting the rooms above the one we had left into bedsits. There was no need for us to slave every hour of the day any more, and we could see we'd had the best years of the small-shop trade. It was soon obvious we weren't going to get much money for the business because corner shops everywhere were suffering from the huge growth of the supermarkets, but it was a relief to think we were going to be without the responsibility.

I was the first to give up, unable to take the stress any more, and to my surprise I discovered, when I went to the jobcentre to sign on, that the office job I had left at Leeds City Council cleansing department was available again. When I went along to see them, I found that many of the people I had known there nearly fifteen years before were still working in the same office. It was like coming back to a family. Things had changed a bit in the office with the introduction of computers – I didn't even know what a mouse was – but the moment I was shown how to work them, I loved it. I had always enjoyed office work and they were a nice crowd of people. My job was called a 'helpline' now, but it was still the same: sorting out people's enquiries about dustbins or rodent control or anything like that. It was such a relief to have a job that didn't take up every hour of the day, and to be able to take a bit of time now and then to chat to other people. I absolutely adored it; it was like going on holiday every day.

Even once both shops had been sold, we still had the bedsits, which gave Keith a bit of an income while he thought about what to do next. It didn't worry me if he never did anything else. He had done enough double shifts in his life to justify an early retirement, although I doubted it would be long before he found something else he wanted to do.

One of the reasons we had to give up the shop was that he had been having recurring trouble with his back and I thought he needed a really decent rest; he'd more than earned it over the years. A few years before we had bought ourselves a really nice bungalow, just along the road from the old one. It had big rooms and plenty of light. We loved it and knew that it would be the perfect place to retire to when we had finally had enough of working altogether.

On 10 October 1995 Matthew rang to tell me he had finished his PhD and was just off to hand it in to his professor. He was twenty-five years old and he had been in full-time education since he was four, but it felt like it had all been worth it. The last time we'd seen him, or heard from him, was a couple of months before, when he'd come up from Leicester to see his aunt, Keith's sister, Colleen, who had come over from Canada on a visit.

'If she's come all the way over from Canada,' he said, 'the least I can do is come up from Leicester.'

We had a big family lunch in Manchester, where Gaynel was living, and our two grandchildren were there – Christian was three and Pippa just one. We loved spending as much time with them as we could, and now that we'd sold the shops we could see them a bit more often. Dena was there too, as well as Matthew. It was great to have everyone together like that. We had a Range Rover at the time, because we needed a big car for going to the cash and carry and other business chores (we called it the Beast because it drank so much petrol), and we dropped Matthew off in town the next day because he was meeting Dena for a coffee at the library café before going home. Keith and I were going to the casino for lunch with Keith's sister and brother-in-law. We had got into the habit of going out for meals during our years in the shops, when we were too tired to cook for ourselves by the time we finished work.

During the visit, Matthew complained about having a toothache, which was unusual for him.

'You must get to the dentist, Matthew,' I said, reverting to the bossy mum role.

'I will, Mum,' he promised. 'I will.'

As Matthew walked away from us that day, we had no idea that it would be the last time we saw him before everything changed.

———

Matthew had three serious girlfriends after Ivona broke up with him. First there was Janet and then, when that relationship finished, he met a very nice girl called Emma, who was also at Sheffield University, although he still stayed friends with Janet.

'I had to stay his friend,' she confided to me one day when she came to visit us after they had split up, 'because he was the love of my life.'

Emma was a lovely, red-haired girl who suffered from narcolepsy, a disease where the sufferer falls fast asleep in unexpected places and can't be woken up. We'd never come across it before and it was a shock to find her on the couch, dead to the world in the middle of the day. Matthew used to joke that he thought it was his conversation that put her to sleep. When she was awake she was a jolly and pleasant girl.

The next girl he brought home was Sarah, whom he had met at Leicester when she was visiting a friend there. She was from a naval family in Portsmouth and she came up to Leicester once she had finished her own degree, moving into the house Matthew was sharing with friends. She was another lovely girl, though I wasn't sure that she was the one for him long-term and I felt that Matthew thought the same. But, as usual, he seemed happy to coast along until the relationship would most likely gradually become just a friendship.

———————

Matthew handed in his PhD as he'd planned; it was 120 or so pages of closely typed material, titled 'An EUV Selected Sample of Selected DA White Dwarfs'. Apparently, according to Matthew, White Dwarfs are 'the most common end stage of non-explosive stellar evolution', whatever that might mean. The next day, Sarah and Matthew went into town to celebrate. They both had some book vouchers to spend and went to the bookshop together. They split up to browse around the shelves, and when they met later they discovered they had both bought the same book.

'Matt didn't eat much that day,' Sarah told me later, 'in fact, I think he'd only had one packet of crisps all day.'

That night they went to a bar and had some drinks. When they came out they walked to the park together and sat around the cenotaph under the autumnal night skies, talking until two in the morning. When they did finally decide to make their way home, they went through an alley behind a row of tall houses that were used by the university as offices.

A metal fire escape ran up the side of the building and Sarah and Matthew decided to climb up it on to the roof, forty feet above, so he could show her the stars. It sounds like the sort of romantic, spur-of-the-moment thing he would suggest. And Matthew had always been a climber, ever since he was a small boy clambering up the wrong side of his bunk bed.

We later saw for ourselves how the roof could be reached. There was a door at the top of the stairs and a sloping roof that you could get across to reach a step on to a dormer window with a flat roof. This bit of roof, high above the ground, was about six feet by six feet, the size of a large double bed.

I can't help replaying the past in my mind, and reworking it so that everything turns out differently. It's a ridiculous game, because we can't change anything that's happened. But all the same, it's tempting to imagine another outcome. I sometimes think that if Matthew hadn't been so clever he would never have gone to university. If he hadn't got a first at Sheffield, he would never have decided to do a PhD. Perhaps he could have chosen somewhere other than Leicester, and done different things and met other people.

If only things had gone differently, that night on the roof would never have happened.

6

Shattering News

At seven o'clock on the morning of 12 October 1995, I was sitting on the sofa in the kitchen of our new home, drinking a cup of black coffee, smoking my first cigarette of the day and gazing into space. I had finished my toast and was lost in a contented daydream, thinking about how well life was going as I prepared myself for the journey to work. The early-morning sun was coming in through the lace curtains and I felt really happy. We'd got rid of the burden of the shops and I was loving my job. All the kids were doing well and Keith and I had

a lovely home. There was nothing more I could ask for.

Keith was still in bed, which was unusual for him. He hadn't yet decided what he wanted to do, and was enjoying the rest from running the shops all those years, with all the enforced early-morning starts. He had kept working there for a while after I went back to work at the council, and I'd helped him out in the evenings after work, but it had been too much and eventually he gave it up entirely. It was wonderful to be free of the responsibility and able to please ourselves in what we did with our spare time.

I saw a figure pass by behind the net curtains, blocking the sunshine for a split second, and then there was a knock on the door. I felt an uneasy stirring in my stomach. Who would be coming round to see us at this hour?

When I opened the door, there was a uniformed policeman standing on the doorstep with a solemn look on his face and my heart gave a horrible lurch. There was no way he was going to be bringing good news at this time of the morning and with a face that serious. My first thought was for the children.

'What's wrong?' I asked, dreading whatever I was going to hear, but impatient to hear it just the same, hoping it wouldn't be as bad as my worst fears.

'There's been an accident,' he said.

'Which one?' I asked, knowing immediately it must be one of the children.

'Matthew. It's very urgent. They've rung through from Leicester but they won't tell me what's happened. He's at the Leicester Royal Infirmary; you need to ring them immediately.' He gave me a telephone number.

The first thing my panicked brain thought was that Matthew had been stabbed. I don't know why it should have been that in particular, but it is the sort of thing you read about happening to young men when they are wandering around cities late at night, possibly a bit the worse for wear from drink. Now I realise that it was much more likely to be a car crash, but I assumed they would have told the policeman if that was the case. My mind raced with scenarios. But what could be so bad that they wouldn't even tell the police what had happened?

Seized with fear, I ran into the bedroom, trying hard not to let the feelings of panic overwhelm me even though I could feel them rushing up, threatening to engulf me.

'Keith, Keith, wake up!' I yelled, shaking him. 'Matt's had an accident. We've got to get to Leicester as quick as possible.'

I was terrified that I was never going to see my son alive again. I remembered him walking away from the car to meet Dena a couple of months before. Was that going to be my last memory of him? It couldn't be true – it just couldn't.

Keith woke up and leapt out of bed at once, hardly able to speak as he processed what I was telling him.

I went to the phone and with shaking fingers I dialled the number the policeman had given me, my mind spinning. It seemed to take for ever to get through to the Leicester Royal Infirmary.

'I'm Matthew Marsh's mother,' I said, my voice trembling with fear and anxiety. 'He's been brought in and we need to know what's happened to him.'

But the person on the other end of the line refused to tell me what was wrong with Matthew. All she said was that we needed to get to the intensive care ward as quickly as we could.

I knew that if it was that urgent that we get to

the hospital, then Matthew might be about to die. It was nearly two hours' drive to Leicester from Middleton, along the M1. There wasn't time to argue with the person on the telephone – we had to get going at once.

'I don't have any money for petrol or food or anything,' Keith said, as he rushed around pulling on his clothes and trying to gather his thoughts. We had never got into the habit of using those holes in the walls of banks because we had always had a float of cash in the shop. We needed cash if we were going to travel that distance. The banks wouldn't be open for a couple of hours yet and we had no credit cards.

Keith ran to the shop, knowing from experience it would already be open, and asked Afsal Ali, who had bought it from us, to lend us something out of the till.

'I'll pay you back as soon as we get back,' he promised.

'Don't worry about it, just get to your son,' Afsal replied. There are a lot of advantages to living in the same area all your life, building up a reputation for being honest and honourable. Everyone round there knew Keith and trusted him. We were so grateful to Afsal – without that money, we wouldn't have been able to get on our way to Leicester as quickly as we did.

I rang the girls but Dena wasn't answering her phone. Gaynel answered though, as she was already up with the children, and she was, of course, shocked and deeply fearful for her brother when we told her what little we knew.

'We're going to Leicester now,' I told her. 'They won't tell us what's happened, just that we need to get there as soon as possible.'

Gaynel knew as well as I did what that meant – Matthew was likely to be on the brink of death.

'You just get there as soon you can, Mum,' she said. 'I'll keep trying Dena until I reach her. I'll join you in Leicester as soon as I can, once I've found someone to look after the kids, OK?'

It was a small comfort to talk to Gaynel, to share our panic with someone who loved Matthew as much as we did, and to know she was going to take care of reaching Dena for us. Once we were on the road we were going to be out of contact because we had no mobile phones in those days. It was an agonising thought, knowing we wouldn't receive any more news, good or bad, until we got to the hospital. The journey was going to seem endless.

Within half an hour of the policeman bringing the news, we were on the motorway, driving at ninety miles an hour, both sobbing, terrified that we were never going to see Matthew alive again, that he might already be dead. I couldn't believe that I had been feeling so happy just half an hour before, or that I had slept through the night without sensing anything was wrong. My child had been in some sort of accident and I hadn't even felt a tremor of his pain. It didn't seem right.

I couldn't stop talking, gabbling with panic about all my fears that Matthew was dead, but I realised that I was making Keith cry more with the things I was saying and that if I wasn't careful we were going to crash the car and never get there at all. I forced myself to be quiet and tried to control my sobs. I wanted to be composed for when I got there, in case Matthew was conscious and needed us to be strong.

That journey is etched on my mind. It seemed endless as we travelled mile after mile of motorway.

Keyed up by our fear and panic, every minute we drove was torturous. The journey seemed to take hours longer than usual. Whenever a signpost appeared on the horizon, I expected it to tell me we were nearly there, but there always seemed to be more miles to go than I could bear. I kept doing calculations in my head, trying to work out how much longer before we got there. Not knowing if Matthew was dead or alive made it impossible to focus my thoughts or prepare myself for what I might have to face. Would I be able to cope if he was already dead? I couldn't think about it. Instead, I focused on our journey: eighty miles to go . . . seventy miles to go . . . On and on it went, endless and agonising.

At last we reached Leicester and found our way to the hospital. We parked the car and then ran in through the doors, desperately asking everyone the way to the intensive care ward. The corridors seemed as interminable as the motorways and the terrible smell of disinfectant closed in around us. Everywhere we looked, there were broken and sick people, some simply exhausted and drained by illness and age. Patients were shuffling around in their dressing gowns and slippers among nurses and doctors with their clipboards and serious, distracted expressions.

At last we found the right place and went to the desk where the nurses were.

'We're Matthew Marsh's parents,' we gasped, out of breath from racing through the hospital. 'What's happened to him? How serious is it?'

We stared about us anxiously, as though we'd see Matthew right there at the desk. It was strange to feel the contrast between our breathless hurry and the quiet, calm atmosphere of the ward.

'Your son is very ill,' they told us. 'He fell off a roof in the night.'

We were stunned. I couldn't take it in. That scene hadn't been one of the many I had played through my head over the previous few hours. I had imagined knife-wielding muggers and drunks with broken bottles. I had pictured speeding cars and a hundred different crashes, but I hadn't envisaged my son falling off a roof. That was the sort of accident that happened to people in broad daylight, people who worked in the world of scaffolding and skips, surely? What was a man on the brink of becoming a Doctor of Astrophysics doing on a roof in the middle of the night? It was all so confusing. I couldn't form any sort of picture that would prepare me for what his injuries might be. Was it a high roof? Had he landed on anything soft? Had he landed on his head? Was he broken beyond repair?

I imagined the horror and fear he must have felt during those few moments of the fall, suspended in the air, waiting to hit the ground. It was hard not to scream out loud at the thought of my child going through that. I wondered if he was instantly unconscious and out of pain when he hit the ground, or whether there were seconds or minutes of agony before he passed out or help came. I felt as if my head was going to burst with so many terrible thoughts clamouring for attention.

'Where's Sarah, his girlfriend?' I asked. I felt she was bound to have been with him, and perhaps she could answer some of the questions already teeming through my brain.

'She's still with the police,' was the reply, which was somehow chilling. The police were involved. This was very serious indeed.

'Where's Matthew?' we begged. 'Can we see him?'

'He was brought into hospital in the early hours of this morning. We've sedated him to relax him and we've kept him unconscious. We'll take you to him now.'

We were led into the intensive care ward, a terribly quiet room full of humming life-support machinery and hushed voices. The patients all lay motionless on their beds, with tubes sticking out of them. They seemed to be in some sort of suspended state halfway between life and death.

Then in one of those beds we found our precious son, also motionless and chillingly absent. Matthew was laid out on a board, because they weren't sure yet what injuries he had to his spine so they wanted to move him as little as possible. I had prepared myself to see him looking battered and broken, but it was just the opposite. He looked the same as ever – the only mark on his face was a small scratch across his nose and he seemed to be sleeping peacefully. He didn't look sick or close to death. It was a strange experience to see him like this – as though we could shake him awake and he would open his eyes and be his old self.

He was connected to a ventilator, which beeped

and purred softly by the bedside, and he was hooked up to other tubes and machines. A nurse was beside him, and we were told that while he was in intensive care a nurse would be there at all times.

A doctor came up to give us a progress report. 'We've given him a scan, and there is a small deformity on his spine. We're not sure whether it's a birth defect or an injury from the fall. So he'll have to stay on the board until we have done some clinical observations on him.'

I was so grateful to all of the medical staff for dealing with a situation where I had no idea what to do. I was so used to always being in control, always being the bossy one who knew what should be done. I could see the fear in Keith's eyes and knew he was feeling as helpless and vulnerable as I was; two strong, capable people who had brought up children and run a business, and we didn't know what to say or where to look. We didn't know if there was something we should be doing or whether we were just getting in everyone's way as they tried to save our son's life. We were completely adrift and terrified of what might be about to happen to our family.

They must have been used to dealing with patients' relatives because they didn't seem to take much notice of us, but let us sit where we needed to be — at Matthew's side. We were asked to wait outside if they were taking X-rays or doing any other procedures, but otherwise we sat with him all the time. Although we were relieved to find he was still alive and we hadn't lost him, our anxiety now came from not knowing what might have been broken or injured in the fall. Was he going to be paralysed? Or brain-damaged? What state would he be in when he woke up? Would he ever wake up? Were they going to need to operate on him? All these thoughts were rushing through our minds as the horribly slow minutes ticked by.

I called my sister, Pat, and Keith's sister, Cath, trying to get my words out without choking on them. I rang Hilda and asked her to pass the shattering news on to Sandra and Rita. I even managed to ring my office and tell them that I would not be coming in to work that day. After we had been there an hour, a policeman arrived and gave us a black bag. Inside it were the clothes Matthew had been wearing when he fell, along with a few possessions like his wallet. The sight of his things made me choke back another sob. I still couldn't believe that my poor boy was lying so defenceless under the crisp white hospital sheets. The policeman had nothing more to tell us. He simply said that they'd come to the conclusion that it had been an accident and there was no need for the police to be further involved.

A little while later, Sarah arrived. She was not hysterical but she was obviously exhausted and deeply shocked and upset at what had happened. She couldn't help but cry when she saw us and she was clearly very concerned for Matthew. She wanted to see him but they were doing tests when she arrived so she sat waiting with us.

'What happened, Sarah?' asked Keith gently. 'How did this happen to Matt?'

'We were looking at the stars together on the roof,' she said. 'I know it was stupid to go up there but it seemed like a good idea at the time. One minute we were gazing at the stars, and then when I turned round, he'd gone. He just slipped away.'

That couldn't be the whole story, I thought. How could he simply slip silently over the side of a roof?

It didn't make sense. But that was all Sarah would say about it, and we didn't want to press her on it. It was an accident and it had happened and that was that. We didn't blame Sarah for anything.

She had to leave for work before we were allowed back in to see Matthew, but she said she would be back as soon as she could. Once again we were on our own, counting the minutes while we waited for some news, praying all the time that it would be good.

None of us know what the future holds for us, not even the next few minutes, but most of the time we are able to forget this terrible uncertainty and fool ourselves that life is predictable and controllable and can be made safe and comfortable. Most of the time it is all those things, but every so often something happens to remind us that actually we are completely at the mercy of the Fates. If something bad is going to happen to you, there is nothing you can do to stop it, and all the plans and certainties you thought you had, about who you were and what your life was going to be like, can vanish in seconds.

We had nothing to do while we waited for the

doctors to carry out more tests and to assess what the damage was. We haunted the waiting areas, looking for places to smoke as we tried to quell our aching nerves and gather our thoughts.

Eventually a nurse came to collect us and took us back to Matthew's bedside where a doctor was waiting.

'Have there been any changes?' I asked anxiously.

'We've had the results of the spinal check,' they said, 'and it turns out that the deformity to Matthew's spine is a birth defect and doesn't need to be corrected. So he can have the board he is resting on removed.'

This tiny fragment of information made us feel like we were moving forward, solving Matthew's problems one small step at a time. Perhaps it wasn't as bad as they had feared at first — perhaps we were going to be the lucky ones, who had a close shave with disaster but came away all right. 'Do you remember when Matthew fell off the roof?' we would say, shaking our heads and laughing. 'That was a narrow escape! He could have been damaged for life.'

Maybe that was going to happen. But then again,

as we stared at our son lying in a coma, his body broken from a forty-foot fall, and the enormity of his accident sunk in, we realised that we were probably fooling ourselves, clutching at straws which would blow away in the wind when they told us the harsh truth about Matthew's future.

'I've washed his hair for him,' the nurse told us, and we knew he would be angry about that when he woke up, because dreadlocks aren't supposed to be washed. But with his clean hair spread out around his head on the pillow he looked so beautiful and so dramatic, like the last of the Mohicans. I didn't know what to do. I just wanted to hug him but didn't dare because of all the tubes and for fear of hurting him. Keith and I were both in shock as we stood helplessly staring down at our only son.

Gaynel and Dena arrived from Leeds before midday and it felt good to know we were all together there for him, that Keith and I weren't completely alone in our grief. Gaynel had driven all the way from Manchester to fetch Dena from the house she was sharing in Leeds. Unable to waken her with the phone or by banging on the door, she had eventually resorted to throwing stones at Dena's bedroom window until she appeared, attracting the attention of a friendly Irish neighbour at the same time.

'Come quickly,' Gaynel shouted up to her bleary-eyed sister when she finally appeared. 'Matt's had an accident!'

A few seconds later Dena had come flying out the door.

'Begorrah,' the old Irishwoman marvelled, 'you've been that quick, are you sure you remembered to put your knickers on?'

They were both in shock, crying and upset but trying to keep calm for all our sakes. The girls were both much better at asking questions of the staff than we were. They knew the right words to use and they weren't in such a paralysed state. They are both such strong characters and they took over for us for a while, leaving Keith and me to sit quietly gathering our thoughts, trying to work out what we should be doing. We felt a long way from home in more ways than one.

All four of us sat around the bed, just staring at Matthew's beautiful, sleeping face, willing him to be all right, not knowing what to say to one another while we endured the endless wait for news from the doctors about his condition.

Later in the afternoon, the girls had to go. Gaynel's children needed picking up from the minder and Dena had to get back to Leeds. They left none the wiser about what was going on inside their brother's head or body, but at least they knew he was still alive and, it seemed, not in imminent danger of dying. We had been given a respite from death, even though we had no idea what life was going to hold for us.

At last, the doctor came to tell us the extent of the physical damage Matthew had suffered. He had broken his pelvis, both at the front and the back, as well as his shoulder blade. He had snapped a few ribs, one of which had punctured his lung, causing him major breathing problems. He had also smashed the ball in his elbow. But he had not broken his back, which was a blessing.

Their main concern when he was brought in by the ambulance had been that his breathing was so laboured; they had decided the best course would be to sedate him, so that he would relax as much as possible. Then they linked him up to a life-support machine to make sure everything continued to function while his body took some time out to heal. The calmer he was, they told us, the easier it would be for his body to recover from the trauma.

'Matthew has been very lucky. There's no major cause for concern,' a senior doctor assured us, once he had told us about Matthew's injuries. 'There are just two or three random bleeds in his head but at this stage we are sure that they're nothing to be unduly worried about. Nothing critical but best to keep him in intensive care for observation.'

That was good to hear. Anxiety still filled every part of my brain, but at least Matthew was alive and looked OK. People with expertise were saying encouraging things, they were giving us reason to hope that soon our ordeal would be over and we would be able to take him home and nurse him back to health. Our initial panic was beginning to subside, replaced instead by a dazed acceptance of this new situation, though we were terribly upset and worried and, I think, still deeply in shock. My overriding feeling was that I didn't want to leave Matthew's side. I wanted to be with him until he was strong enough to look after himself again. I didn't know what I could do to help, but I knew I couldn't walk away and leave him there alone.

But how could we stay with him when we lived so far away? I didn't want to be a two-hour drive away from him. What if he came round and none of his family was there? What if he suddenly got worse? I couldn't face that agonising two-hour dash back again.

'As long as he's in intensive care, we can give you a room to stay in at the hospital,' the staff told us.

It was wonderful news and we were so grateful for their kindness. We were completely in their hands. They showed us to a little room with two beds and a basin, which looked as if it would serve us very well while we were there. The main thing was that we were going to be close to Matthew, on hand at any hour of the day or night in case something happened. In our dreams, it would be him waking up and asking for us. In our nightmares, it would be his condition deteriorating for some reason. Whatever, it was an enormous relief to know that we didn't have to trek back to Leeds, and that we could be near our son in his darkest hour.

7

Cabbage

From the moment that we saw our temporary living quarters, our lives fell into a new pattern. Our previously secure and well-ordered world had disappeared — it was like a dream, a fading memory, a life that had been lived by someone else. Instead, over the next few days, the sounds and sights and routines of the hospital ward became our new world. The whirl of strange faces that had greeted us when we first arrived began to become familiar, but familiarity did not bring any comfort.

As hour after hour passed, with no change in

Matthew's condition, we began to accept our new reality. How was it possible that we had been so happy and so optimistic just a few days ago? Our home, with all its privacy, security and comfort, might as well have been a million miles away. We had lived in the same area all our lives, the homes we had moved between had been only roads apart from each other. We knew our own place and we belonged there – but now we were suddenly living in someone else's universe and everything was different. We felt we didn't belong there, that the hospital had nothing to do with us apart from the fact that our son was on one of its wards, and it didn't seem to care that we were there. There was nothing of us, or our past, in our little room, no possessions, no photographs, no memories. It was just a place where our bodies slept. And the unfamiliarity of our surroundings only made us feel all the more consumed by our anxiety.

Our day-to-day reality was no longer getting up, making breakfast, going to work, chatting quietly, making dinner, watching telly and going to bed. Now the only thing we knew was sitting at Matthew's bedside, clinging to the hope the doctor had given us that there was 'nothing to be unduly worried about', waiting for the whole ordeal to be over so we could go back to the world we had known all our lives.

More than anything we longed for Matthew to be back with us. We wanted him to open his eyes and talk to us, so that we knew he was fighting to recover his strength. But he just kept on sleeping.

The next news we had was that the only operation the doctors wanted to do was to wire together Matthew's shattered elbow.

'There's nothing we can do about the breaks in his pelvis,' the orthopaedic surgeon told us as we sat outside the ward. 'But don't worry, it'll mend itself over time, as will the shoulder blade and ribs. He may not exactly be walking about right away, but we're positive he'll be up on his feet in due course. And we're planning to rouse him from his sedation in three days.'

Three days didn't sound so bad, compared with the pictures we had been conjuring up in our imaginations of Matthew locked in his coma for months or even years. Our hopes flared up once more. If they woke Matthew up in three days and thought that he would soon be walking around, there could be no great harm done. He would probably be back to something like his normal life after some more weeks of rest and recuperation. Keith and I kept telling one another these things, to keep our own spirits up as much as the other person's.

Everything seemed to be about waiting, or sleeping in the tiny room we had been allocated. Often we would pass some of the waiting time by going out for cigarette breaks, relieving the monotony and tension with long walks down what seemed like miles of sterilised corridors to the fresh air.

Over the next few days, Sarah came every evening, Gaynel and Dena came when they could, and several of our friends from home visited, having driven down from Leeds to be with us, providing us with the moral support we needed so desperately. It was reassuring to see familiar faces and hear friendly voices, reminding us that our world was continuing and that we had only stepped out of it temporarily. They would all still be there when we went back, when the nightmare was over.

The operation went ahead and we waited – something we were getting very used to – smoking incessantly to calm our nerves until the news came through that Matthew was out of the theatre. The surgeon was very happy with the way everything had gone, full of optimism. The operation had been a success and we were another step forward. Next, they told us they were going to bring him out of his coma, just as they had proposed days earlier.

The big day arrived. We had been watching Matthew lying unconscious without any change for several days now. It was very exciting to think that he would soon be back with us. I couldn't wait to talk to him, to tell him how much we loved him and how worried we had been. The doctors had all been so encouraging and optimistic about Matthew's chances of recovery, that I was sure we would be soon be chatting away like old times.

We watched and waited as the doctors stopped the drugs that had been keeping Matthew in his unconscious state, so that he could begin to come back to us.

As he started to return from wherever he had been towards consciousness, Keith saw Matthew begin to bite down hard on the tube going into his mouth, the one that went down his throat to deliver his air. At once he knew something was badly wrong and then we watched in horror as Matthew's left arm and left leg shot upwards in involuntary spasms, curling up, useless and helpless. Immediately, the nurses tried to unbend them, but his muscles were as solid and unyielding as iron bars.

We both stood there stunned, knowing this was a terrible sign. The doctors immediately readministered the drugs, and Matthew sunk back to unconsciousness. Their expressions were no longer full of optimism, but grave, as they gave us their new diagnosis.

This new development, they told us sombrely, was evidence of spasticity. They didn't explain any further and I was profoundly shocked. I know now that it is a medical term, meaning that Matthew's muscles were affected by spasm and paralysis, but at the time, I heard terrible echoes of school playground taunts and saw visions of Matthew twisted and helpless. What did it mean for him? Was he going to be like this permanently? Could these involuntary muscle spasms be cured, and if so, how?

Or would he for ever be bent over like some over-grown foetus?

There was a mood of deep concern in the room that Keith and I found terrifying.

'It means he has suffered a brain injury,' the doctor told us quietly. I think that he was disappointed too.

All the hope and optimism we had been nurturing so carefully drained away in a split second. Our wonderful, brilliant son was brain-damaged? He wasn't going to be coming back to us as they had promised, walking about within a few weeks, putting this dreadful experience behind him?

Matthew's mind, the doctor explained, should be telling all his muscles to relax, but it wasn't, and this was very bad news indeed in the circumstances. Nothing on the brain scan they had done when he was first admitted had warned them this would happen. The only evidence they had of what must have gone wrong inside Matthew's head was what we could all now see happening in front of our eyes. Matthew's arm and leg were bent up tight, locked into position, forced to do what his damaged brain was telling them.

They immediately wheeled him away to do another brain scan. When they came back they told us that the damage had now become 'diffused', although we didn't know what that meant.

Then we were called to a meeting with the senior doctor and the intensive care nurse. We were frightened at this new development, and utterly confused about what it meant for Matthew.

It was now that we were delivered the most crushing blow of all.

'Your son will be a cabbage for the rest of his life,' the senior doctor told us, 'or a vegetable, or whatever you want to call him.'

I want to call him Matthew! I screamed silently. But no words came out.

———

Keith and I walked away from that meeting in profound shock. We had been told that our brilliant, beautiful, popular son had no future, that he was condemned to life as a creature who barely existed. We had been advised to put him in a home and forget him. We had been told that, all along, there had been no hope, no dream of recovery. Our visions of Matthew talking to us, walking about, getting better, going on with his normal life had been mirages. They would never happen.

'He will never change,' the doctor had said, and a great darkness engulfed us. As parents, our hearts broke.

He had recommended that we walk away from our son and go on with our lives.

As though Matthew had never existed, and didn't continue to exist? Did he have no idea of what this felt like, and what it meant? There was never even a second's doubt in my mind: we would never walk away from Matthew, or any of our children. It simply wasn't feasible.

But, in the deep uncertainty and heartbreak of that moment, I wished for something else. I wished he would die.

I know that sounds awful, and seems to run counter to what any parent would want for their child. But, in the despair of that day, I saw a terrible future for Matthew and I couldn't bear the thought of him going through it. I saw a terrible future for all of us, as we lived with and cared for the pale shadow of himself that Matthew had become, being cruelly reminded every day of what both we and he had lost. As his strong young limbs withered and aged, and his life slid by without him being aware of it and without any of the experiences and possibilities he had dreamed of, it would be an ongoing punishment that none of us deserved.

More than that, I knew I wouldn't have the strength to be the one to nurse and care for him in that state – it was simply beyond my capabilities.

At that moment I had no idea how we were going to cope with the future – the thought of abandoning him to the care of strangers when he was so helpless and vulnerable and unable to protect himself was unbearable. Even though the future was so uncertain, I don't think many parents could understand how at that moment I wished my son dead.

8

The Awful Reality

When the doctors tried once more to rouse Matthew from his coma, the same thing happened: he bit down hard on his air tube, cutting off his vital supply. So they stopped trying to wake him, and instead allowed him to slip back into the peaceful coma they had disturbed him from, so he could wake from it naturally when his system was ready.

There he lay in his hospital bed, unconscious, just as he had been when we arrived — but now there was a terrible difference. The sight of his twisted, locked limbs was a painful reminder to us all that his mind was injured and had shut down, perhaps for ever.

I couldn't believe that after all the strenuous efforts the medics had made to save Matthew's life over the previous few days, they were now willing to write him off so easily and completely. Now I wished with all my heart they had let him slip away on the night of the accident so that we did not have to carry on suffering like this. I knew that Matthew would never have wanted to be a vegetable in a home somewhere. When he had been home in August, Matthew and Dena had watched a television programme together about Anthony Bland, a victim of the Hillsborough football disaster in 1989. Anthony was seventeen years old when he went to the match and, trapped by the panicking crowd, he was one of the victims crushed so badly his chest caved in and his lungs collapsed, cutting off his oxygen supply. His cerebral cortex was destroyed within minutes. Four years later he still lay in hospital, fed by tubes, the part of his brain that should have provided him with consciousness turned to fluid. The High Court had decided that it would be right to withdraw the feeding tubes and allow him to die peacefully.

Dena and Matthew had both agreed that they would not want to live under those circumstances. Who would? And now, just months later, Matthew was actually in that same position. Would he still want the same thing — to be allowed to die, as Anthony Bland had? Or would he want us to keep hoping for a miracle?

As we sat at his bedside, it was so hard to keep from buckling under the despair. We had never cried so much in our lives. From the moment we heard about the accident, Keith and I wept bitterly all the time, as though the floodgates had been opened after a lifetime of controlling our emotions. Not a day of our hospital vigil went by when we weren't overcome with overwhelming despair. Partly we were crying at our own helplessness: a parent always wants to be able to make things right for their children, even when they are old enough and smart enough to be the ones doing the caring. But we were being told that there was nothing we could do for our boy; there wasn't anything anyone could do apart from make his body comfortable for as long as he continued to breathe and his heart continued to beat.

Matthew's life, as we knew it, was over. That was the message we had received from the medical staff, the doctors and the experts. But we couldn't grieve his loss because he was still technically alive, lying in front of us, asleep. It felt like being trapped in hell with no chance of ever escaping.

After a lifetime of always being in control of everything that happened around me I suddenly found myself powerless. It should have made me feel humble and grateful to everyone who tried to help, but instead I felt frustrated and angry. I was angry with Fate for making this happen to us, and I was angry with the doctors who had first led us on with false hope, and then abandoned us to utter despair. It was hard to remember how I had ever felt light-hearted enough to be able to dance for hours on end, or what it was like to laugh. Until that moment I had enjoyed such a happy, carefree life: spoiled as a child, loved by a wonderful husband, blessed with beautiful, hard-working children. I had never had to face anything like this before. During the days, sitting beside Matthew's bed, I would force myself to smile all the time, and at night, in the privacy of my bed, I would sob myself to sleep. I was strained to breaking point but, for Matthew's sake, I had to stay strong and keep going.

Although we had no idea what we were going to do in the long run, in the short term we knew we could not just walk away and leave Matthew to the care of strangers, however well educated and experienced they might be. As long as he was in the hospital, we would stay there with him. Whatever happened afterwards – and whatever it was, it would not be abandoning him in a home somewhere – we would face when that came along. For now, we were committed to being with our son and making sure he was comfortable and cared for.

From the moment that Matthew was declared a hopeless case, it felt as though the hospital authorities and staff saw Keith and me as a nuisance. No longer were we the agonised parents of a desperately sick boy; now we were in-the-way, besotted parents who weren't able to accept and come to terms with the inevitable. It was as if they had turned off the tap that had poured out all the encouragement in the first days; now they just wanted us to accept what they were saying and step aside to let them, the professionals, do their job. We were surplus to requirements, unwanted guests who had outstayed their welcome.

The person who was kindest to us as we struggled to come to terms with the emotional tidal wave that had hit us was the cleaning lady on the ward, who showed us a little room where the doctors made themselves coffee and tea, so we could boil up a kettle from time to time and make ourselves something hot to drink. It was easy to forget, when there were so many critically ill people around us, that our own systems were under stress as well. Beset with anxiety, neither of us were eating or sleeping much. We just smoked and worried. Every morning we would be up at seven and straight in to see our beloved son, then downstairs to wait patiently for the canteen to open, before we spent another day just going through the motions of sitting by his bed waiting for him to wake up.

We were completely out of our depth and we couldn't find the right words to express what we were feeling or to ask the right questions. Keith told the consultant that Gaynel and Dena wanted to talk to him, knowing that they would be able to make more sense of what was going on than we could, but for one reason or another the consultant was always too busy to see them. I guess our girls can be quite scary when they're angry; they are both very forthright in their views, just like their parents, only with the education to back their arguments up.

The girls refused to give up — we needed some answers to our questions. Eventually they managed to get one of the junior doctors to explain about the two scans of Matthew's brain. They wanted to know what the difference was, and why the doctors now believed that the damage was 'diffused'.

The young doctor told them that there wasn't much difference between the two scans. In fact, from the things he said to Gaynel and Dena, they realised that the doctors' prognosis of Matthew's future was based on the way his body had reacted to being wakened, rather than the scans. But there was no more explanation than that.

Now that the surgeons had mended Matthew's elbow, there were no more operations they could do. They hadn't changed their minds on that one. His pelvis and shoulder blade would mend themselves, as would his ribs. His lung, which had ripped itself free of its mooring in some places and so had contracted, was also mending, although it was now restricted in size.

'People survive perfectly well on one lung,' they assured us. 'His breathing won't be a problem.'

I wasn't too happy about that, remembering how Matthew used to suffer from hay fever in the summer months as a child, sometimes getting it so badly it turned into asthma. But a little difficulty with breathing was nothing compared to the problems we now knew he had in his head.

The longer we stayed around the ward listening to the doctors and nurses, the more medical information we picked up. The more we watched, the more it seemed to us that they didn't really know what to do with him. Knowing what I do now about brain injuries, I realise that every case is different and often it is a matter of reacting to what the patient needs as and when he needs it. But even so, as far as we were concerned as parents, no one could have a greater capacity to care for Matthew than we did. We became determined not to leave him in the care of others.

I was still silently praying that Matthew would die and be spared this life of complete dependency that they were now all quite certain he was headed for. Just as I had believed the experts when they said there was no cause for concern, I now believed them when they said there was no hope of him ever recovering. I knew he'd had a wonderful life and I thought it would be so much better if it ended now. To have lived as full, happy and active a twenty-five years as Matthew had done was more than many people ever achieved. What would be the point of him continuing for another fifty if he knew nothing about it and had no way of enjoying his life?

But Keith never thought like that and, over the next few days, as we sat beside our son's bed, watching him sleep, he began to think things through more logically and less emotionally. He was always better than me at keeping a cool head in a crisis. How could we write Matthew's future off so easily? he wondered. If the doctors had been able to change their minds once, why couldn't they change the prognosis again at some future date?

After all, we'd been given the wrong impression initially when we'd been reassured that there was no cause for undue concern. They weren't always right, by any means.

They seemed very sure that the damage was irreversible. But what if they were wrong?

The doctors still didn't even know exactly what damage had been done inside Matthew's head, although they thought it must have been an impact of the brain against the inside of his skull since there was no sign of a blow on the outside. Keith was beginning to realise that, where brain damage was concerned, very few outcomes could really be predicted. Just because one prognosis said that Matthew would never recover, he reasoned, didn't make it a fact.

While I was sitting there, willing Matthew to give up the struggle and slip peacefully away, Keith was willing him to fight his way back to health. He didn't want to lose his son.

9

Counting Our Blessings

A few nights after we had been told Matthew would never recover, I was sitting on my own beside the bed while Keith was taking a cigarette break, when the staff brought in a man who was a victim in a car crash.

There were about six of his relatives standing around the bed, keeping vigil while he died, looking bewildered and lost. When I heard that he'd gone I felt so happy for him, and envious of those people who were now mourning. They were all crying for their loss, but all I kept thinking was how lucky they were to be able to grieve for their loved one, to have been given an ending, a conclusion. How much easier that would be, I thought, than being left hanging in limbo.

If Matthew died then, in his sleep at that moment, I reasoned, he would never have to suffer again. From the moment he fell and hit the ground he had been unconscious, so if he never woke up he would know nothing about it. It seemed like a much kinder fate than the one they told me now lay in store for him. Losing him would be terrible for us, but he would feel no pain and no sadness, and we could let our tears flow like the relatives at the other end of the ward. All the worry, anxiety and uncertainty would be gone and we would be free to concentrate on our grief.

I doubt if losing a child ever becomes bearable for any parent, whatever age that child might be. It is not natural to have your children die before you. Even if you're in your nineties and they're in their seventies, I am sure it is still the most terrible thing that can befall anyone. If what the doctors predicted was true, though, for me Matthew was already dead. We had already lost him and actual death was a technicality, a mere ceasing of a heart-beat.

As I sat by the quiet bedside, looking down at my poor boy, I thought of what it would be like if he died. How would I cope with the pain? Then I thought of a way I might be able to dull it, at least for part of the time. When Keith's sister, Colleen, had moved to Canada in 1957, because travel was so expensive in those days, her parents only saw her once more before they died. So, I decided, if Matthew died, I would tell myself that he had moved to Canada, and that he couldn't afford to come back to see us. That, I told myself, was how I would deal with the loss, by fooling myself that it was just a temporary separation. When he didn't ring me on birthdays or at Christmas, I would mourn him for a while, then I would go back to pretending he was living in another part of the world. I can see why so many people down the ages have liked to believe there is a heaven, so they could imagine they were going to one day be reunited with lost loved ones. I've never been devout and I didn't have the luxury of that belief, so I would have to try to trick my brain into believing something different. But I reasoned that at least this way I would cry only twice a year, instead of every day.

I don't know how well my scheme would have worked; probably it would have allowed me peace of mind some of the time, with terrible moments of remembering and having to accept the awful truth that he had gone for ever and that we would never see him again. But I believe that even this would be better than seeing his body in a home twice a year, when the personality that was Matthew had died just as surely as if his heart had stopped beating.

'Just go in peace, Matthew,' I whispered to myself, over and over again, as if he could hear what was little more than a thought.

The next day Keith and I were outside having a cigarette break and we got talking to a young girl of twenty-five who was in the hospital because she had tried to commit suicide.

'I can only remember ever having one happy day in my whole life,' she told me, and I thought that

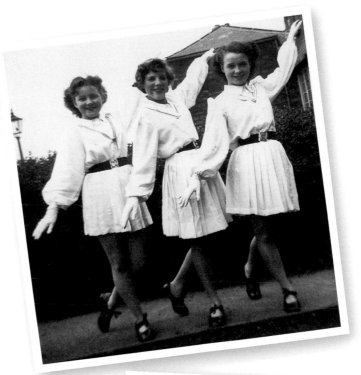

Above, left to right: Sandra, Mavis & Hilda dancing to Bell Bottom Blues in 1954.

Mavis & Keith, Blackpool, 1958.

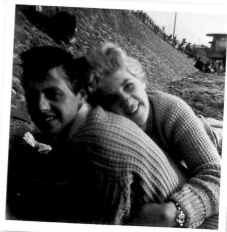

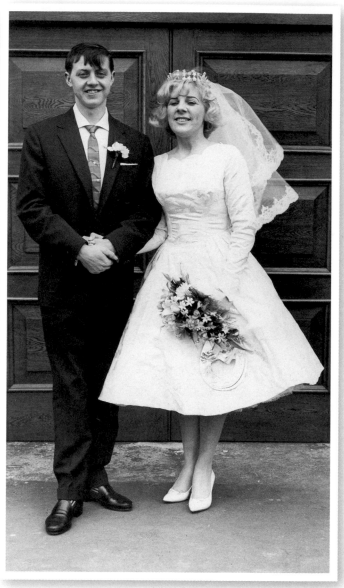

Mavis & Keith on their wedding day, 26th March 1960.

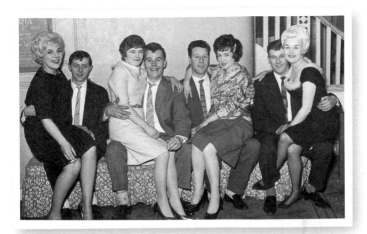

At the Ibbotsons dance, February 1961.
Left to right: Mavis & Keith, Rita & Arthur, Bill & Hilda,
Barrie & Sandra.

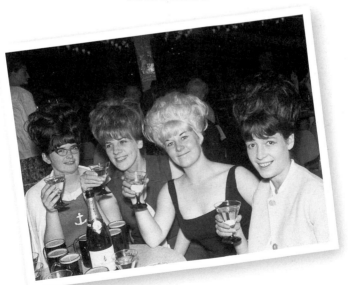

'The Girls' with their bouffant hair-dos on a night out dancing, 1962.
Left to right: Rita, Mavis, Sandra & Hilda.

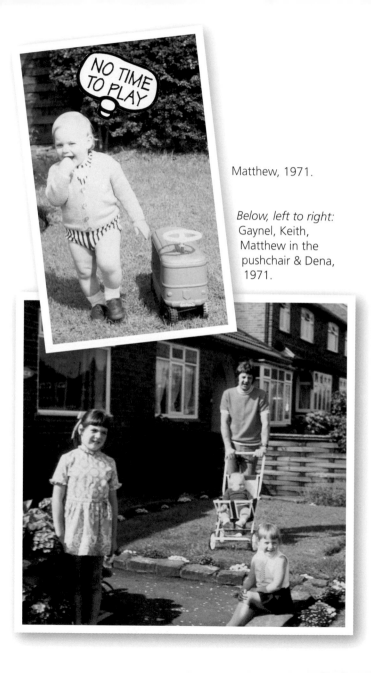

Matthew, 1971.

Below, left to right: Gaynel, Keith, Matthew in the pushchair & Dena, 1971.

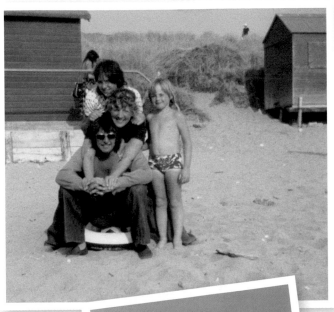

Above: Gaynel,
Mavis, Keith
& Matthew,
Cornwall, 1975.

Dena & Matthew,
1975.

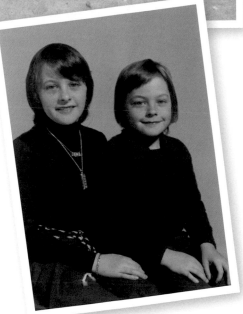

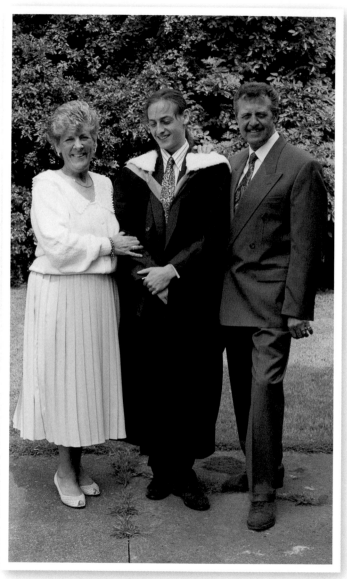

Mavis, Matthew & Keith on Matthew's Graduation Day,
Sheffield University, June 1991.

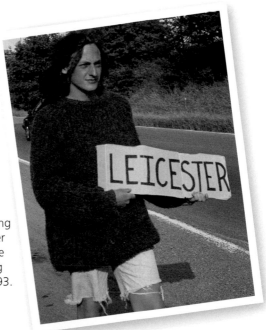

Matthew heading back to Leicester University where he was studying for his PhD, 1993.

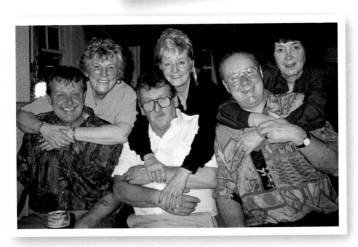

Left to right: Keith & Mavis, Barrie & Sandra, Bill & Hilda, November 1994.

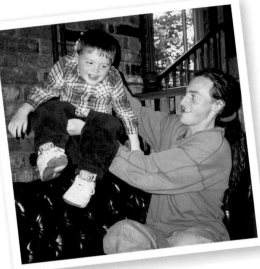

Matthew playing with his nephew, Christian, August 1995.

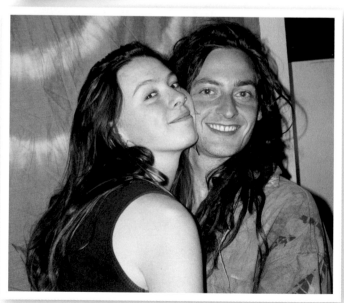

Matthew & Sarah, the girlfriend who was with him when the accident happened.

if Matthew died that night at least he had had twenty-five happy years. I felt so sorry for her.

'You go back out there and change your life from now on,' I gently advised her. 'Make it happy. You're young and fit, so you just enjoy your life and don't let people hurt you any more.'

She asked for a cigarette and I gave her one as we went back in to renew our bedside vigil. Maybe that wasn't the best thing to give her in the circumstances, but we had come to rely on our cigarettes for comfort even more than we usually did, and I guessed she was the same. Needing a smoke gave us an excuse to come out of the room regularly, and something else to think about. Some nights we would be sitting beside Matthew's bed until midnight. We would finally decide to go to our little room for some sleep, but on the way we would invariably have one last cigarette, never wanting to face lying in bed awake, our thoughts churning over and over in our heads. We would make the long walk out to the smoking area and would stand in the moonlight, huddled against the cold, trying to drag a few last moments of comfort from the tobacco as the tips of our cigarettes glowed in the gloom and we talked over the day's small events for the hundredth time.

Our chat with the young suicidal girl showed me that I was learning to be more patient with other people's problems than I had been at the start of our stay there. When we first arrived, my temper was short and if I heard someone in the hospital complaining about something petty I would boil up with indignation, thinking how much luckier they were than us and how they should appreciate their good fortune.

Gaynel and Dena were visiting as often as they were able, and it was Dena who pointed out to me that you can't compare people's problems like that. Their troubles were just as real to them as ours were to us. No doubt there were other people who were worse off than we were and who would think we were lucky for what we had got.

I tried to be as positive as I could, even though it was difficult under the circumstances. There were so many hours of just sitting, staring at Matthew, and we had so much time to think but only one thing on our minds. I tried to come up with some blessings I could count, to try to make the whole nightmare seem less unbearable, and surprised myself by managing to come up with quite a few.

For a start I could thank God this hadn't happened to my friend Hilda or my sister Patricia, both of whom only had one child; at least we still had the girls to think about and put our hopes in. I was also really grateful that we already lived in a bungalow so if we were ever able to take Matthew home, as Keith was now determined we would do, we wouldn't have to find the money for expensive alterations, or to move house. Another blessing was that we had sold the business the year before, so Keith was going to be able to dedicate his days to Matthew for as long as necessary and we had the rents from the bedsits and my job to keep us afloat. If the accident had happened while we were still running the shops I don't know what we would have done. We would just have had to put the shutters up at the windows and abandon our business, I suppose. We would never have been able to run the business and be at the hospital a hundred miles away.

We were also lucky that the girls were grown up and we didn't have anyone else we had to look after.

I could hardly imagine how hard it must be for people who have a child in a situation like Matthew's but have to leave them because they have jobs and other children to take care of. We were fortunate that we were free to dedicate ourselves to Matthew's recovery for as long as he needed us.

I was also grateful that Keith and I were together. I could see that some of the parents coming in to visit the patients were without partners, either because they were bereaved or divorced, and I thought how much harder it would be to cope with the physical and emotional strains if you didn't have someone you loved to talk to and lean on, someone who felt the same as you and understood exactly what you were going through. Even if you had married again, the stepmother or stepfather would never be able to experience quite the same feelings as the biological parents, I'm sure of that.

We heard a lot of stories in the coming years of how the stress of having a head-injured child had split couples up. So many marriages are walking a fine line anyway and the emotional and physical strains of having to care for a damaged child can often be the final straw, particularly if the parents have different ways of coping with their worries and sadness. Our case was, I am thankful to say, very different. We needed each other so much that, if anything, Keith and I were being cemented even more firmly together by what we were going through, despite the fact that we had very opposing opinions about the best outcome.

We had been together more than most couples, having met so young and spent so many years working side by side in the shop. We both knew exactly how the other thought, and how they were likely to react under pressure. So the situation wasn't giving either of us any nasty surprises about each other.

By the time we came back into the warmth of the corridors after our midnight breaks, we would want to take one last look at Matthew before we turned in, like nervous new parents peeking in at their slumbering baby, fearful that he might have stopped breathing in our absence, wanting to have one last look at his sleeping face before leaving him to the care of the nurses and the machinery for a few hours.

We knew we were getting on the nerves of the

nursing staff but it wasn't something we could afford to care about. We simply could not tear ourselves away from his bedside for more than a few minutes at a time. We were always looking out for something to happen: I hoped that he might pass peacefully away, while Keith clung to the hope that we would see some sign of a miracle break-through. We couldn't bear the thought that, if Matthew did wake up, he might find himself alone. So we were a constant presence in the intensive care ward.

Staff in hospitals must look back longingly to the times when visitors were only allowed in for an hour or two a day. In those days a matron or staff nurse was a figure of authority, someone who would expect to have her orders obeyed by mere members of the public. But just as the power of the priests and the teachers has waned since our youth, so has the power of the hospital tyrants. It was good that we now all felt able to be with our loved one as much as we needed, and that we were able to ask questions and challenge the old assumptions. With that freedom, though, came a responsibility to do the right thing, and neither Keith nor I had any idea what the right thing now was. It would have been quite comforting to have been able to put our trust in some all-powerful matron or consultant, believing they had all the answers.

On Matthew's fifth day in intensive care, I was back beside his bed, where I sat nearly all the time, when I sensed someone wanting to get past me to the door. I moved back to let them by, but there was no one there. Then it came again – a very strong sense of a presence behind that I had to let pass. I have never had any sort of religious or spiritual experience, but it felt to me as though someone had just brushed past me. It was such a strong physical sensation and I couldn't fight the impulse to move, even though I could see nothing.

I wonder if that's Matthew, was the thought that popped immediately into my mind. I had the clearest sense of a physical presence that wanted my attention. Was this, I wondered, Matthew's way of telling me that he wanted to live? Perhaps he had felt me urging him to pass on, and needed to tell me that he wasn't going to give up like that. I know that when you are tired and under intense emotional strain the brain plays strange tricks – all your senses are heightened and your mind is suggestible — but the presence felt very real to me.

I was so affected by this experience that I immediately changed my mind about Matthew dying. I no longer wanted him to go. Instead, I joined Keith in wanting to make him better, and vowed to do whatever I could to help. We would show them, and now I knew Matthew was fighting too.

10

Blocked Pathways

We quickly became used to being with Matthew all day, stroking his head and squeezing his fingers to remind him that we were there. His sisters were often with him as well, coming down to Leicester every few days and sitting by his bedside. Friends and family visited too, and it was a great relief to have their support.

Sarah also came frequently to visit Matthew. We were always glad to see her and we knew she was a nice girl who meant a lot to Matthew. We just wished she would feel able to tell us what had happened on the night in more detail, but it was obviously painful and embarrassing for her. None of us could find the right words to say in order to find out more when it was all still so recent and upsetting for Sarah. She had told us that when the police took her in for questioning after the accident they had put a lot of pressure on her, as if trying to catch her out in a lie. On the strength of her statement, they had decided not to look into the incident any further and I certainly didn't want to unnecessarily question her any more than the police had, even though I did want to know more. The police report from the night Matthew was found, which we weren't shown until much later, described evidence that suggested the accident may have occurred while he and Sarah were having sex. I couldn't really understand why they would be doing that on a roof at that hour of the morning when they had a house to go to with a comfortable bed, but I suppose it would have been quite romantic lying under the night sky like that, if a bit chilly at three in the morning.

All Sarah had said in her statement was that they were looking at the stars together and when she turned round he had slipped away, just as she had said to us. The memories of that night must have been difficult for her to deal with, and I could understand why she might want to block them out of her consciousness in order to be able to cope with them, but I wished she could remember more details to tell us. I wanted to understand exactly how all this had happened. I could understand, though, why she found it hard to talk about. But it seemed, in many ways, such a preventable accident and I needed to know how it had come about. Maybe, I thought, if Matthew did come back to life, he would be able to explain to us what had gone wrong on that night, how he had come to lose his balance so badly.

It was our friend the cleaner who suggested that we gave Sarah a bit of time alone with him. In our minds, Matthew had reverted to being our baby and we had become so single-minded in our support of him that we'd forgotten that he'd had another life on the day he had fallen, somewhere a hundred miles away from us, among people we didn't really know.

When it finally dawned on us, with the help of the cleaner, that Sarah needed some time alone with Matthew, Keith and I took the opportunity to walk around the town and have a coffee. It was good for us to have a break from the stifling atmosphere of the ward, but we didn't really know what to do with ourselves when we weren't with Matthew. He was all we thought about and all we talked about every waking moment of our days. We were just killing time when we were away from him, unable to do or think about anything else, and I couldn't help but feel on edge, worrying that something might be happening at the hospital and we couldn't be contacted. I wanted to be there if he woke up and needed me – and I wanted to be there if something worse happened.

Eventually we couldn't bear wandering aimlessly around any longer and made our way back. Matthew was just the same as he had been when we had left.

A few days after the accident, Keith asked Sarah to take us to the building where it had happened. We stood there for a while, staring at the place where this momentous event had occurred. For some reason, I wanted to take a picture of it, and as I took the photograph, I saw that there was a car parked in the spot where Matthew had fallen. I couldn't help thinking that if that car had been parked there on that night, it might have broken Matthew's fall and saved him from this devastating outcome. Perhaps he would have broken a bone or two, but at least he wouldn't have been this unconscious person whose future looked unimaginably bleak.

All I could do as I stared up was to try and understand — why had it happened? Why had they gone up there? I felt so confused that such a small, random decision could have such consequences. It all seemed so stupid and pointless. But there were no answers. We could only return to the hospital and try our best to look forward, rather than back.

———————

To help him breathe as he slept, Matthew had a tube down his throat. Because he kept biting down on it whenever the medical staff tried to bring him a bit closer to the surface of consciousness, they decided they would have to give him a tracheotomy, which meant making a hole at the base of his throat and inserting the tube through there. He also had a tube going into his stomach to keep him nourished until he was able to start eating again for himself, if he ever was able to do that. Using that, they were able to feed him a disgusting-looking liquidised slush, pretty much like baby food. I suppose that is more or less what all food looks like by the time we have chewed and swallowed it.

The nurses gave us the paperwork that went with the feeding tube, in case we decided to take him home to look after rather than putting him in an institution. Reading it over, I saw that the document said that the tube was 'for life'. Those two words hit me hard. The thought of Matthew never being able to have food in his mouth again was very upsetting. Like Keith, I was now absolutely refusing to accept that this was what was going to happen. Our son had to wake up and he had to regain at least some of his faculties in order to live a worthwhile life. We couldn't allow Matthew to be a cabbage, it just wasn't an acceptable option. We had to find a way to feed him properly so he could enjoy tastes and flavours again. It was part of being alive, surely.

———

Although we were becoming accustomed to living in a hospital environment, and learning more all the time about what went on there, it was still a frightening and confusing place. We didn't under-stand much of what was going on around us. Medical staff were always so busy and they talked to one another in what seemed to us like a private language, full of words that meant nothing at all. Some of it sounded alarming and occasionally we would think we had understood something that seemed hopeful, but we could never be sure. We didn't know what questions to ask, or what devel-opments we should be worrying about. In our fear and confusion, and our eagerness to protect our son and make him well, we probably came across as aggressive and abrupt with the staff on many occasions. We knew that but we weren't able to change, at least I wasn't.

Keith is a much more patient person than I am. He always has been. But even he lost his temper once or twice, exploding with frustration when he just couldn't get the staff to understand what Matthew needed. Even though he was generally much calmer and quieter than me, I think even his persistence was getting on their nerves. The fact that we were always there seemed to annoy them. When patients are on their own and trapped in their beds, they are not in a strong position to make any demands, but if they have an able-bodied person with them who is not afraid to speak up on their behalf, the balance of power in the ward becomes disturbed.

On the whole, we understood that the staff were busy and pressured and didn't have the time to explain things to us, but looking back now I wonder if maybe they didn't really know what was happening either and didn't want us to realise. We all expect our doctors to know everything, but of course they often don't. Now and then one of them would be able to give us an explanation that we could understand and our knowledge would increase by another small measure.

'Imagine a bomb has hit the centre of a city,' one doctor said, trying to explain what he thought was going on in Matthew's head. 'You go up one road and you aren't able to get through because it's blocked by fallen buildings. So you try turning left but you meet another pile of rubble. That is what has happened in Matthew's brain; the signals are still there and they are trying to get through, but they are having to find new pathways because the existing ones are damaged and blocked by swelling. They'll keep trying to get a new pathway through to the next connection and it's possible some of them will eventually find a way through. All the cognitive abilities, like being able to speak and make your limbs obey your commands, happen on the periphery of the brain, a long way from the centre, which is why the messages are having such trouble getting through.'

He went on to explain that after the first forty-eight hours the swelling would have started to go down, which was why they had kept him sedated to begin with, keeping him stable to give the brain as much time as possible to heal. Sometimes, he explained, they were able to operate to relieve the pressure but they didn't think they could do that with Matthew. We read later that having a hole drilled into the skull can sometimes lead to a patient experiencing fits afterwards, so I'm glad they didn't go down that route.

On the sixth day after the accident they decided he was no longer in danger of dying, and they moved him out of intensive care into a high-dependency ward. They were cleaning the ward that he was moving to, so we had to wait outside with Matthew as he lay on his trolley bed. Sarah was with us on a visit and overheard a conversation between two of the nurses, which Keith and I weren't listening to, having got used to tuning out most of what went on around us unless we thought it directly affected Matthew.

Something they said made Sarah obviously concerned, and she turned to them and asked suddenly, 'Do you have MRSA here, then?'

The term meant nothing to Keith and me at that time because there still hadn't been anything in the media about the deadly infection that was spreading through hospitals at the time, but Sarah was a biologist and knew a bit more about these things than we did.

'Do you know what MRSA is?' one of the nurses asked, looking a little guilty, as if she had been caught out in an indiscretion.

'Of course I do,' Sarah said, but she didn't go any further, not wanting to alarm us any more than we already were, so the moment just slipped by, like so many others. It was just one more thing we didn't understand. All we knew was they changed their minds about putting him in the main ward and moved him on to a separate room on his own. It was a while before we realised that he had been isolated because he was going into a sort of quarantine. We learned much later that Matthew had indeed contracted MRSA and they were isolating him in order to stem the spread of the infection.

There were so many aspects to Matthew's care that I would never have been able to predict, knowing nothing about it until we actually had to go through the experience. When a body goes into a coma, it needs to have a lot of maintenance work done to it, so that it is fit to function if or when the coma finally ends. Matthew had to have special boots fitted, for instance, which were like braces made of foam and straps, designed to hold his feet at right angles to his ankles, otherwise there was a danger his tendons would tighten through lack of use and his feet would become stretched out as if pointed so he would never be able to sit up comfortably with his feet flat in a wheelchair. Each day he had to be turned over every two hours, be washed and have his teeth cleaned, have his waste bags emptied, food and liquid bags replenished, the tubes into his body cleaned, and physiotherapy to keep his muscles in shape. If a body is getting no exercise or movement at all the muscles will just waste away through lack of use. Physiotherapists have to keep things moving for at least a few minutes every day.

It was a complicated routine but after a while, it was as familiar to us as a working day. We knew what would happen when, and why. It was all designed to keep Matthew's body ticking over, so that it stayed as healthy and fit as possible.

Although we were delighted that Matthew was out of intensive care, and that his life was out of danger, there was an immediate repercussion that we hadn't foreseen. As soon as he left intensive care, we were told we had to vacate the little room we had been living in for the previous two weeks, without being offered any alternative. We had dashed back to Leeds once or twice during the time we'd been in the hospital to get more money to cover all the meals, drinks and cigarettes we were having to buy, and so we already knew we couldn't commute back and forth each day. It was awful to spend even those few hours away from Matthew and we drove far too fast up and down the motorway as a result.

It was a blow to lose our little room, which might have been impersonal and small, but at least provided us with a bolt-hole close to Matthew. We knew it wasn't feasible for us to drive home every night but we didn't want to rent anything in Leicester or go to a hotel, so for the first couple of nights we got a few hours' sleep on waiting-room couches around the hospital, curling up on anything we could find, like passengers stranded at an airport. We had become refugees and I can understand now why those crowds of displaced people you see on the news always look as if they are sleepwalking through their lives. We were so disoriented by everything that we didn't know if we were coming or going, and even making simple decisions like where to stay became an overwhelming problem. In a way, we were thrust back to that state of shock we had experienced when we first arrived as we wandered about, sleep-deprived and ill at ease.

None of the staff seemed to notice that we were drifting around like lost souls. Their priority is the patients, I suppose, not the shell-shocked relatives who are too desperate to be near their loved one to leave the premises, even if it means sleeping on hard hospital chairs.

Thinking about those early days and weeks now, I can see how much we needed help as well. Just as soldiers and policemen need counselling when they have witnessed horrific scenes, the close relatives of accident victims often need caring for. But like everything, I suppose, it is all a question of cost and time — it might be that looking after relatives would adversely affect the care given to the patients themselves. Even so, I still think that there could have been someone there to check that we were coping and to advise us on our options, rather than letting us live like virtual vagrants around the hospital premises.

We slept rough in the hospital for two nights, going home once to have baths and pick up changes of clothes. But we couldn't risk staying away from the hospital for a minute longer than we had to, fearing something would happen while we weren't there.

Then we remembered that Matthew's room in the house he had been sharing with four others, including Sarah, was empty and we slept there one night. Sarah had gone home to her parents by then to recover from the shock of the accident. It was very hard being in his room, among his belongings. It smelled of him and reminded us of how he had been little more than a fortnight before, making our hearts ache. I have never experienced pain like I felt that night. Mothers are always affected by the smells of their children — I suppose it's some primitive instinct designed to help them recognise their own offspring. I know that if a farmer wants a ewe who has lost a lamb to adopt an orphaned one, they will skin the dead lamb and wrap the skin around the living one, to fool the ewe into wanting to take care of it and feed it. Smells are so important and I'm sure one of the things that is so unsettling about being in hospital is that all the natural aromas are wiped out by the overpowering antiseptics and disinfectants.

It was good to have somewhere comfortable and friendly to go to sleep, but the emotional cost was too high. The pain of being constantly reminded of the contrast between the old Matthew who was no longer in his room among his possessions and memories, and the silent, sleeping body in the hospital bed was too much to bear and we didn't go back.

As the days went by the news of what was happening inside Matthew's head didn't get any better, although we hardly ever understood what the doctors were telling us when they described their latest findings. They told us, for instance, that they had done tests and measured him on something they called the 'Glasgow Coma Scale' (GCS), which tests a brain-injured patient's response to pain, and assesses the level of eye-opening and verbal response. It is scored between 3 and 15, and Matthew was less than 8 which indicates severe brain damage. Was that what they meant when they said he would be a cabbage? Vegetables have no senses; they can't enjoy anything in the world around them. Was that what it was going to be like for Matthew if he ever woke up?

Keith believed that he would wake up, and would return to normal, and I was struggling so hard to share that optimism. Sometimes it was impossible to imagine how we were ever going to be able to give him back even a part of the life he had lost.

The physical evidence that we could see with our

own eyes was equally depressing. His muscles had become so taut in his left arm and leg, his fist clenched so tightly as it pressed into his cheek, that he was doing himself injuries, even as he slept. It was like watching a baby curled up in pain, and being unable to reach out to provide relief. The longer he stayed unconscious, they told us, the worse the damage was likely to be when, and if, he ever finally woke up.

It was terrible to look at Matthew lying there and to know that time was running out for him. Soon, he would never be able to recover his physical fitness. With each day that passed with his muscles still locked in position, the journey he was going on risked becoming too long for him ever to turn back.

'Wake up, Matthew,' we begged him, sometimes silently and sometimes aloud. 'Wake up. Come back to us. Please.'

11

Matthew's World

Matthew's friends from the university started to come in every day once he was out of intensive care, sometimes as many as six at a time, and sat around the bed talking to him and about him as if he were a conscious part of the group. For us, it was a wonderful distraction from our own gloomy company, but we were mainly pleased for Matthew. We'd been told that it was possible he could hear what was going on around him, even if he wasn't able to respond, so we liked the idea of there being voices that might be familiar to him, talking about happy things, rather than just the worried voices of his parents and the businesslike tones of the nurses and doctors.

We had never met any of these people before, only the ones he had brought home as girlfriends. They all came from his four years in Leicester, although some of them were only in the first or second years of their courses. They were visitors from Matthew's other world, one that we had known nothing about until now. Just as they knew nothing of the memories we had of his childhood, we knew nothing of their shared experiences beyond what we were learning now. It was a different world to ours, one where he had been an adult man with adult interests and friendships, not just someone's son or brother. Meeting these young people and listening to them talk about Matthew was like eavesdropping about someone we hardly knew.

It was an eerie feeling to be reminded that our son had had this separate existence while we had been going on with our lives back in Middleton, and it was moving to discover how well liked he was by everyone who knew him. One friend told us how Matthew always used to advise people to 'go for a walk in the woods' when they felt life was getting on top of them. It was just the sort of advice I could imagine him giving. A French girl told us how she had arrived in Leicester with nowhere to stay and he had given up his bed for her, staying in Sarah's room until the girl was able to arrange something for herself.

They all talked about his patience and good nature, his sense of humour. They reminded us how he had never been a good timekeeper, always refusing to wear a watch, and several remarked on his liking for a pint of Guinness. His professor, and head of department, Martin Barstow, admitted that he had been a bit taken aback by Matthew's long dreadlocks when he first saw him.

'He looked like one of those eco campaigners who used to hang around in trees to stop bypasses being built in areas of natural beauty,' he said. 'I hadn't encountered a PhD student like him before. He was always quite laid-back in his approach to finishing work, so I had to push him a bit more than some students to keep things ticking over.'

Later he admitted he did have some worries about how Matthew would do in the job market. 'I wasn't sure if he could project himself enough to get a job in astronomy, where you need to be quite aggressive to get on. This disadvantages people who are basically as nice as Matthew.'

I liked to hear that Matthew had done so well, despite being a bit casual about the work, and that the only thing his professor thought might hold him back later was the fact that he was too nice. That sounded like a pretty good character reference to me.

I kept a visitors' book in Matthew's room, so that whenever someone called in to see him they could leave a note for him. My hope was that when he woke up, he'd be able to read all the entries and see who'd been round to check on him.

A lot of people left messages for him to read, so he would know he was never forgotten by his friends. They were all so positive and friendly and lacking in any of the embarrassment or awkwardness that older people sometimes feel when they are in hospitals; they gave Keith and me a much-needed injection of youthful optimism.

I was hoping to find out more about what happened on the day of the accident, but none of them seemed to know anything, although the professor remembered how he heard about Matthew's accident.

'I was in the middle of carrying out a thesis exam for another student when the postgraduate tutor phoned me with the bad news,' he said. 'I was stunned, but I had to carry on with the exam. The student was actually a friend of Matthew's so I couldn't say anything for fear of undermining the exam.'

Despite the fact that we were beginning to make new friends in Leicester, Keith and I knew that all the travelling to and from the hospital every time we needed to get money or clean clothes was too much of a strain for us. Then my sister Pat made a brilliant suggestion – why didn't we get Matthew moved from Leicester to the Leeds Infirmary?

It made complete sense, so we asked the doctors if they would move him to Leeds now that his condition had stabilised, so he would be closer to home. It seemed quite possible that he would be in hospital for months and we didn't think we could cope with being so far from home for so long. We were hopeful that this was a reasonable request but what felt like the usual negativity was the response. It couldn't be done. It was impossible. There was no way that Matthew could be moved somewhere better for his family, because there was no room at Leeds Infirmary.

It seemed unlikely that such a big hospital could be so full it couldn't take one critically ill patient whose family lived in the area. Pat wasn't willing to be fobbed off so easily and wrote to a local councillor, pointing out that if the hospital denied us what seemed like a reasonable request, it was very likely that there was going to be another accident with us driving up and down the motorway all the time in such a state of exhaustion and shock. Our situation must have made sense to someone objective on the outside and I suspect the councillor pulled some strings, because a couple of days later, we were told that Leicester

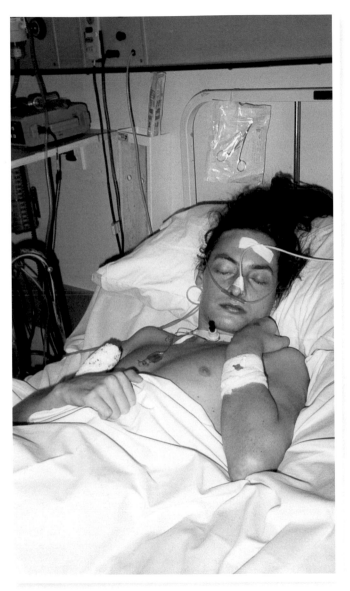

Matthew in Leeds Infirmary after the accident, November 1995.

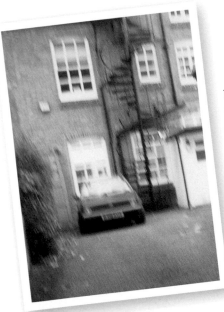

The scene of Matthew's accident. The car is parked where Matthew fell, and the fire escape stairs to the right is how he and Sarah reached the roof.

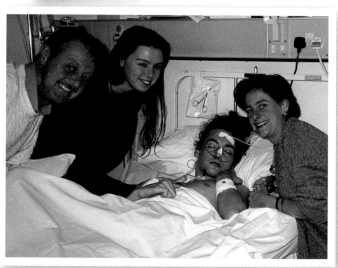

Keith, Sarah & Dena visiting Matthew at Leeds Infirmary, November 1995.

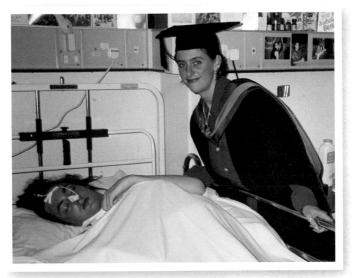

Dena visiting Matthew on her Graduation Day, November 1995.

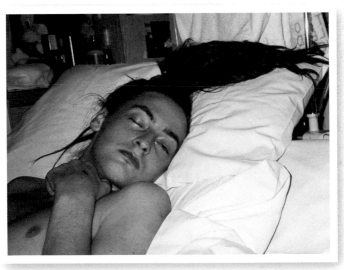

Three months after the accident, Matthew is still in a coma, but has opened one eye slightly. Leeds Infirmary, January 1996.

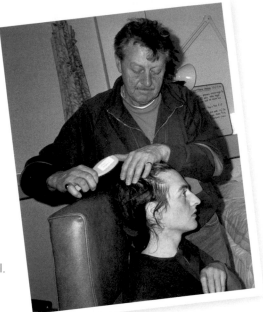

Matthew has woken from his coma, March 1996. Keith did everything he could for Matthew whilst he was in hospital.

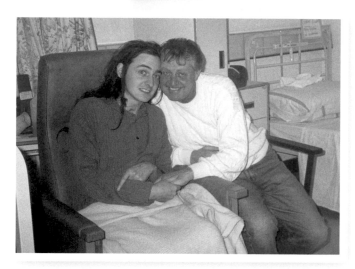

Matthew & Keith, 'always together', March 1996.

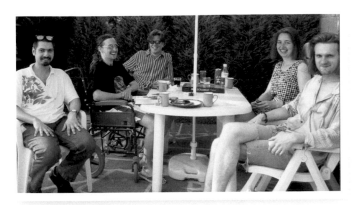

Matthew with his friends from Sheffield University, 1996.

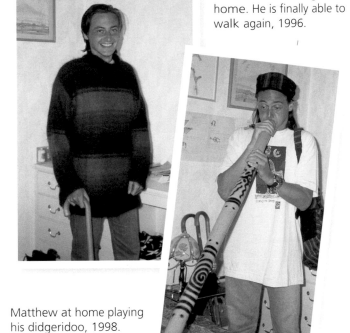

Matthew recovering at home. He is finally able to walk again, 1996.

Matthew at home playing his didgeridoo, 1998.

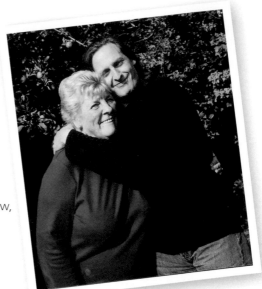

Mavis & Matthew, 1999.

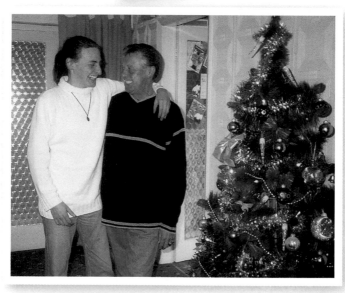

Matthew & Keith, Christmas 1999.

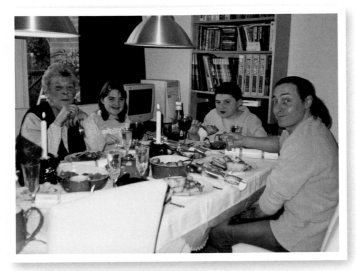

Christmas lunch, 2003. *Left to right:* Mavis, Philippa, Christian & Matthew.

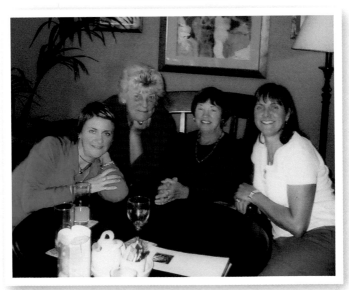

Left to right: Dena, Mavis, Auntie Colleen & Gaynel.

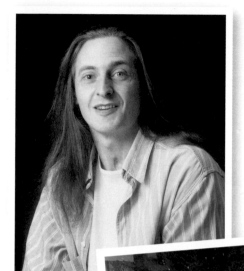

Matthew, February 2001.

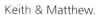

Keith & Matthew.

Royal Infirmary had agreed to move Matthew to Leeds and there was no more talk of there being no room.

By now, it was three weeks since Matthew had fallen from the roof, but it felt more like three years. Our past lives and everything in them seemed like a distant memory.

The transfer was arranged. Sarah came to see Matthew off from Leicester, overseeing his loading into the ambulance, while Dena and Keith waited for him at the Leeds hospital. I was at home, catching up on my chores while I waited to hear that he had arrived safely.

As soon as Matthew reached Leeds Infirmary, they did some tests, discovered that he had MRSA and put him straight into a side room to isolate him from the other patients. For the first time we were told that Matthew had this infection and something of what it meant. Suddenly the conversation we had half heard between Sarah and the nurses made sense. I sometimes wonder if it was the reason the doctors at Leicester were not keen to have Matthew moved to another hospital – perhaps they didn't want the bug to spread and hoped that it would clear up before anyone else heard about it. Perhaps they didn't want other hospitals to know that MRSA was active in Leicester.

Dena said the doctors in Leeds told her Matthew was in a terrible state, with thrush on his genitals and in his mouth, although Leicester had told them he was clear of any infection. The doctors at Leeds later told us they believed Matthew should never have been allowed to move in that condition and that it risked spreading the infection to another hospital. In a selfish way, I'm glad it was not mentioned, or we could have been trapped in Leicester for weeks.

Keith and I were not panicked by Matthew's new setback. For one thing, we knew hardly anything about MRSA as it wasn't widely known about at that time, so we didn't realise how serious it could be. For another, we had a strange confidence that Matthew was going to come through, and even this infection didn't shake our faith. It was just one more challenge in the huge battle for Matthew's recovery.

When I realised that Matthew was riddled with infection, I thought back to how many people the hospital in Leicester had allowed to be crammed into his room at any one time, and shuddered. Sometimes the room had been so crowded with friends and relatives I'd had to come out for air, so any bugs in there must have been having a field day.

Now that Matthew was openly diagnosed as having MRSA, we all had to take extra precautions when we entered and left his room. We now understood just how important it was to avoid the infection spreading to any of the other patients, having read up about it. In 1995, the general public still weren't really aware of how quickly this bug was spreading through the hospitals and the official line was that it could be contained if we were all careful. Every time we went into Matthew's room we had to put on disposable gloves, taking them off and throwing them away when we came out. The trouble was, Keith and I were constantly going in and out every half-hour through the day for our cigarette breaks.

'Do you realise you've used a whole box of gloves?' a nurse told me crossly on the second day as we headed back outside yet again. 'We can't have this.'

In my strained state, it was very easy to lose my temper and I did so now.

'Tough,' I snapped. 'Get another box of bloody gloves.' Which was a lot politer than the words going through my head. By that stage I was approaching the end of my tether and I didn't take kindly to being given lectures about something like latex gloves. It seemed like a small thing in the bigger picture. I was willing to buy a box of latex gloves myself if it was going to be such a contentious issue.

It's certainly true that it would have been much better to give up smoking, but I can say without a doubt that this was not the time to start trying. Those who say we should have exercised more willpower perhaps don't understand that it's hard enough to give up smoking when you have no troubles and stresses in your life. In those desperate days, cigarettes provided a comfort in our hour of need. If we hadn't been able to smoke at such a stressful time, I don't know how we would have held up.

———————

It was a great relief that Matthew was now so close to home. It meant we could sleep every night in our own bed and eat proper home-cooked meals again. It was lovely to be able to spend evenings at home and to be able to do simple things, like clean the house, do the washing and then iron the clean laundry. It eased a lot of pressure on us and meant we had some escape from the hospital; we were able to talk and cry in privacy at night while we waited for sleep to release us from the anxieties of each day. It was a tiny step back towards our old lives, but only a tiny one.

———————

Right from the start, the doctors had told us that the first sense to come back to someone in a coma is their hearing, so we were warned always to be careful what we said when we were near to Matthew, in case he was taking it in. It's sometimes hard to remember that when you have been sitting for weeks beside someone who gives every appearance of being asleep, but we were being pretty good about it.

Dena was in Matthew's room on her own and a doctor came in to check on the patient. He was a handsome sort of fellow and a bit full of himself. Standing right over the bed, just a few feet from Matthew's head, this doctor said, 'He's got the worst form of MRSA. There's only one sort of antibiotic we can use.'

'So what are you saying?' Dena asked, her hackles already rising.

'If the head injury doesn't kill him,' the doctor went on blithely, 'the MRSA probably will.'

'Don't talk like that over my brother,' Dena said. 'If you want to say something like that, you take me outside to tell me.'

When I met the same doctor later, he said ruefully, 'I don't think your daughter likes me.'

'I don't think it's you,' I said. 'It's what you said.'

Quite often we saw doctors forgetting to put gloves on when they came in and then going on to see the next patient, although I was always quick to remind them, which didn't please them. They liked to be the ones dishing out the tellings-off, not the ones receiving them. I probably should have been gentler with everyone around me and more diplomatic, but I have always been a forthright woman and I can't stop myself from blurting out what's on my mind. I couldn't understand how they thought they were going to stop the spread of MRSA if they were going to be so careless in their practices.

The MRSA was adding to our worries. Matthew had small wounds on his hand and chest where the tubes had gone in that just wouldn't heal and I hardly dared to think what would happen if he caught any more infections. There are inevitably so many germs flying around in hospitals, and if a patient's immune system is ceasing to function, they are constantly at risk.

I used to put Germolene on Matthew's cuts each night, a product we had known and trusted all our lives, but I knew it was a futile little gesture, and unlikely to make any difference. It was frightening to think that something had got into his body that was stopping it from healing. During our lifetimes we have grown used to thinking that antibiotics and antiseptics will cure everything, forgetting that only a hundred years ago people would routinely die from the smallest infections. We had grown to believe those times would never come back, but now they seemed to be returning for Matthew.

One weekend morning when Keith and I came into the ward together, after he had been at Leeds for four weeks, we could see immediately that the staff were all really excited about something. For a wonderful moment we thought perhaps he had woken up, maybe he was even up and walking about.

'It's gone,' they told us.

'What's gone?'

'The MRSA. We can't understand why, but it's just vanished. He's completely clear. We can't believe it. It was the worst strain possible to have and he's clear.'

'There you are,' I said to Keith, only half joking, 'I told you that Germolene was good stuff.'

It was a wonderful moment but we didn't dance about with joy – for one thing, we'd never really realised how dangerous the infection was. Of course it was amazing that it had simply disappeared, and a great step forward, but in a way I was disappointed that I hadn't come in to find Matthew up and about, which was all I dreamed of. And I'd always been confident that he would beat the infection. It was just a small step on his larger journey.

―――――――

Once Matthew was clear of MRSA, he was moved out of his isolation and on to a ward. Leeds Infirmary is a wonderful hospital and Matthew's early treatment there was superb. But once he was on the ward, the nurse who had been dedicated to his care became a nurse who also had to look after a lot of other patients. It meant that it was impossible for Matthew to get the kind of care and attention that we felt he needed. Because we were always confident about speaking our minds when we saw what we believed to be bad nursing practices, willing to contradict them or disagree if we thought they were wrong, we found our popularity quickly diminishing. We grew increasingly horrified by the amount of time nurses stood around talking, or sat doing paperwork, when patients needed help. More often than not, it was easier to do the jobs ourselves than to try to get nurses to do them.

A sign over Matthew's bed said that he should be turned every two hours. This was to avoid bedsores, and if we knew he needed turning, we would remind the nurses, which drove them mad.

'We'll be with you in a minute,' was all they ever said. Whenever any patient or relative asked for anything they always got the same answers. It was similar to the negativity we had experienced in Leicester. No one ever said, 'Sure, OK, let's do it.' There was always something else more important that had to be done first. I am sure there were occasions when there were other, more important things to be done, but because it was always the same reply, it often seemed as though they had got into the habit of saying it. Perhaps the nurses felt that they should not respond to our requests immediately or they would never hear the end of them. It made me frustrated because it was not my idea to turn Matthew every two hours — there was a sign over his bed that said he needed it, so when the time had passed, we could hardly pretend it didn't matter.

If they still didn't come after they had promised, we would turn him ourselves. But I was constantly terrified that Keith would damage his back again through lifting Matthew — who was quite a weight in his unconscious state even though he was shrinking down from his usual ten and a half stone to nearer seven — and I would be left to cope on my own at Matthew's bedside.

As we sat day in and day out in a hospital ward, we saw some unsettling things. We would watch as meals were put down in front of patients who were incapable of reaching that far, or of lifting the food to their mouths. When the orderlies returned and found the food uneaten they would simply assume it wasn't wanted and take it away without stopping to find out why. It seemed to me that there were people in there who were being given nothing to eat all day sometimes, simply because they were not able to protest or do anything to help themselves. Sometimes I wasn't able to stop myself from speaking out and our popularity continued to sink.

The physiotherapists were great, and we watched everything they did like hawks, thinking that we might one day have to do this for Matthew ourselves. It might soon be us working on the slumbering muscles to make sure they didn't waste away before he woke up and started using them again himself, if he ever did wake up. Dena would come in with her aromatherapy oils and would massage his face, arms, hands or his feet, which looked so gnarled and uncomfortable, for hours on end, keeping him moving, soothing and healing, talking to him all the time, letting him know that he was being loved and cared for. I had no idea if she was right about the healing powers of using aromatherapy, but I was sure the feel of her fingers, the sound of her voice and the loving attention would do him good. I believed it might reach through the coma to something deep inside him that was still awake and listening to what was going on outside his motionless body.

Often it was the non-medical staff who were the most helpful and considerate, like the cleaner in Leicester who had told us where to make tea and coffee. There was a young girl who handed round the food who told Keith he could go into the fridge whenever he wanted.

'I've left you a little orange juice in there,' she said.

Keith would get a sponge and soak some orange into it, then dab it on Matthew's tongue just to moisten it and give him some flavour to think about. He might be getting all the nutrition he needed through the tube in his stomach, but we instinctively felt his mouth and throat needed to be stimulated and used. Keith did the same with some soups and ice creams. Even though Matthew was unconscious his throat muscles seemed to respond to the moisture and flavours.

'You can't do that,' a nurse scolded when she saw what he was doing. 'He could choke on that with the tube in his throat.'

'I'll take that risk,' Keith replied, because by that time we had been in the hospital long enough to no longer be intimidated by the medical staff with their rules. We were beginning to find the courage to make our own decisions about some things, to know what chances were worth taking in order to make Matthew's life a bit more comfortable. At times we even had to fight for his rights. When we were told he was going to miss a Friday session of physio, for instance, because they didn't have enough people on duty, we insisted someone came in at the weekend to make sure he didn't go too long without movement. If we hadn't been there, he would have been left, because other people were. We knew that the physios were doing their best and were over-worked and unable to get round to everyone, but our priority was to keep Matthew as fit as possible, ready for when, or if, he opened his eyes and returned to us. We couldn't afford not to be single-minded. We couldn't afford to worry about whether we were annoying other people or treading on their professional toes. Our son was all that mattered.

As the weeks passed, Keith became really good at doing everything for Matthew: turning him every two hours so he didn't get bedsores, cleaning him up when he had messed himself, or suctioning his ventilator tubes when they got blocked so that he could breathe more easily. He learned everything from watching the nurses and doctors.

No wonder nurses are so busy. Even with just one patient, there always seemed to be something that needed doing. Matthew was wearing nappies again, just like a baby, and when he smelled something funny, Keith would roll up his sleeves, get a basin of soapy water and get on with it. The nurses would usually poke their heads round the curtains to ask if they could help, just as he was putting Matthew back into his pyjamas and settling him down.

'Everything all right, Mr Marsh?' they would chirp.

'Just changing him,' Keith would say.

'Oh, you should have called us, we'd have done that.'

'Not to worry, love,' he would smile grimly. 'You're busy. I can do it. I've nowt else to do.'

Actually Keith was quite happy to do it all — it was better than just sitting there knowing Matthew was lying in dirty nappies for hours, waiting for someone to have time to see to him. Although we were driving the nurses mad, I guess there must have been times when they were quite glad of the help. Keith was so much better than me at keeping his temper at times like that. I was never able to hold my tongue and my popularity with the staff was, not surprisingly, low.

But it wasn't just us who were seeing all these things going on. On one occasion, the drip that was putting fluids into Matthew's body started making his arm swell. Keith and I weren't there at the time, but Keith's sister, Cath, was visiting and noticed the arm beginning to balloon. She watched for a bit, to make sure she wasn't imagining it, and then called a nurse. As usual the nurse promised she would 'come in a minute'. When she did eventually get to the bed, she realised that instead of the drip going into Matthew's vein, it was going into his muscle. I dread to think how long it would have been before anyone had noticed if Cath hadn't been there.

Sarah told us that she was going to be giving up her room in the house in Leicester. It wasn't surprising since there wasn't anything to keep her there now that Matthew was back in Leeds. She also told us that other students were wanting to move in and it was obvious now that Matthew wouldn't be going back there in the near future, so his room would have to be emptied. Gaynel and Keith drove down to pack up and bring all his belongings back home.

While they were away, I was sitting with Matthew on my own when I noticed blood oozing out of his mouth. I became worried and asked a nurse to have a look for me.

'That's quite a common thing,' she assured me, having taken a cursory glance. 'When people lie in a coma for a long time their gums start to bleed. Don't worry.'

By the time Keith came in three hours later, having driven all the way to and from Leicester to fetch Matthew's belongings, he was shocked to see the blood. I told him what the nurse had said and asked him to have a look and see what he thought. He gently prised Matthew's jaw open and peered inside.

'It looks like clots of blood to me,' I said. 'There's too much of it to be just coming from the gums.'

Keith was not in a patient mood, having been driving all day, and he called out to a doctor, 'Hey, you, come here! There are clots in here. It looks like he's bitten his tongue. This isn't good nursing.'

For a moment it looked as if the doctor was

going to remonstrate with Keith for his angry tone, but he came over anyway and looked inside Matthew's mouth. He had to agree and set about cleaning it up. Again, I hate to think how bad things would have to have got before the nurses had thought to do anything themselves.

———————

That evening I had the sad task of putting all Matthew's things away in his bedroom at home, sniffing his clothes as I folded them into drawers and remembering how he had been just a few weeks before. In one shoebox I found every letter he had ever received while he was away at university, all neatly filed in their envelopes. After each new find I had to sit on the edge of the bed and wait for the tears to subside before I could continue. As I stacked his books on to his shelves I found five foreign dictionaries: Spanish, French, Polish, Italian and German. He also had *The Selfish Gene* by Richard Dawkins and *A Life in Science* by Richard Feynman. There were too many for the shelves to hold and I had to put some in other bookcases around the house. I rested his guitar beside his bed and set up his stereo and television. I put his juggling balls into a large wicker basket and asked Keith to fasten the wind chime to the ceiling when he came home later that night. Now it was all ready for our son to return to, when he finally got better. We could only keep praying that he would.

12

Struggling On

It was a health worker who first suggested to us that we should sue the university for the accident. The idea had never occurred to me because I had always been one of those people who doesn't believe in the compensation culture. Accidents happen in life and if you go round taking people to court you just end up making things worse. Everyone from the university had been so kind to Matthew, both when he was conscious and now that he was in a coma. I didn't think it would be right to start accusing them of being negligent, but I listened anyway.

'How can we sue anyone?' I asked. 'It was his own fault for being up on the roof in the first place. He had no business being there.'

'It's not up to you to decide that,' the health worker said. 'It's up to the law. Matthew was at the top of his field; he would have made a good living. If you can find any fault and you can just get a small percentage of that for him it might be a fair amount of money. It might help to look after him in the future.'

It seems to me that the readiness of everyone to sue is one of the things wrong with the modern medical system, making all the doctors and nurses spend their time covering their backs, and I felt similarly about the university. But at the same time I had been starting to worry about how we would afford to buy all the things Matthew might need in order to live out a comfortable life once he was no longer being looked after by the hospital. It was impossible to know at that stage just how handicapped he was going to be, and I knew how expensive it was to look after someone full-time. As long as Keith and I were alive, we could work to give him everything he needed. But what would happen once we'd gone? Or if Keith became ill or hurt his back and I wasn't strong enough to lift Matthew on my own? I didn't think it was fair that the responsibility should all fall on Gaynel and Dena if it was possible to get some insurance to help. Just because we were content to spend the rest of our lives nursing Matthew if it proved necessary, we could hardly expect them to do the same, and how would they be able to afford to pay for the help they might need in years to come? The number of different potential problems I could imagine developing once I spent some time thinking about it made me feel physically sick with worry.

Although I didn't feel completely happy about it, I went to see the firm of solicitors that the health worker recommended. It made me feel as if I was money-grabbing, as if I was trying to put a price on Matthew's life, and I didn't like that.

Once the solicitors found out about Matthew and the potential seriousness of the problem, the most senior man in the practice said he would like to handle the case himself. He listened carefully as I described everything that had happened and said he needed to talk to Sarah in order to assess whether or not there might be grounds for a claim.

Sarah very kindly came up to Leeds to talk to him and he rang me a few days later.

'I'm sorry,' he said. 'I don't think you have a case. If there had been a slate missing or some faulty guttering, maybe we could have made a claim. But it doesn't seem that the university was at fault here.'

I was disappointed that Matthew wouldn't have a little money to help him through whatever lay ahead in the coming years, but in a way I was relieved, because I had never truly believed he was due anything. If we had got anything, I would have felt we had won it under false pretences in some way, even if we had never done anything except tell the truth. If an adult is daft enough to climb up on to a roof in the middle of the night, after having a few drinks, and then starts messing around, how can anyone else be held responsible if he loses his balance and falls off? It wouldn't have been right.

But the question still remained: how would Matthew be looked after once Keith and I had gone if he remained as damaged as they predicted? Even if he was only partially handicapped, how would he manage? There seemed to be so many things to worry about that I could hardly remember what it must have been like that morning a few weeks before when I had been sitting in the sunny kitchen, thinking how happy my life was.

Occasionally we would get glimpses of our old life, like when Dena graduated at a ceremony in Leeds Town Hall that November. All of us were gathered there to watch her being honoured, just a hundred yards from the hospital where Matthew was lying unconscious, completely unaware of how the rest of his family were spending the day.

As the weeks went past, we began to think in more practical terms about the future. If Matthew was going to need a lot of nursing, we had to make sure we still had some money coming in. We had got used to the idea that we had only the two of us to support for the rest of our lives, which was why it had not seemed a problem to give up the shop and slow down on the way towards our retirement. But now we had to accept that Matthew had become our responsibility again. That meant that at least one of us needed to get back to work. As I was the one who already had a job, and since Keith was much better at dealing with nurses and doctors than I was, we decided I should go back to work during the day, and then come in to the hospital to join him and Matthew in the evenings. Six weeks after the accident, I went back to my job – my employers had been very understanding and kind about letting me take the time I needed to be with Matthew.

It was a punishing schedule though. Sometimes we wouldn't go home until midnight and I would feel so tired, having been up since seven in the morning. One late night when we got to the Range Rover we found it had a flat tyre. Poor Keith had to change it in the freezing cold, with snow on the ground. I felt so sorry for him after he had spent so many hours nursing Matthew without a word of complaint, but I was too tired myself to be able to do anything to help. I just sat watching him from inside the cold car, feeling completely useless.

Despite the exhaustion of working and visiting the hospital, I was glad to be back at work. It lifted my sprits and it was a relief to get a change of scene and to have something else to think about. I still loved my job and the distractions of a busy office would work for hours at a time, helping me to forget about the nightmare that had consumed our lives. But every so often a picture of Matthew would come to my mind and the sadness would overwhelm me again. Then I would have to go outside for a smoke and a little cry in the cold fresh air, before I was able to pull myself together again and get on with things. I don't know if I would have held up as well as Keith if I hadn't been able to escape for those few hours every day.

The only reason I could leave Matthew at all was that I knew that Keith was with him all the time. I trusted him completely to look after our son and to do the right thing, more than I could have trusted myself, in fact. I had always known he was a lovely man and a great husband and father, but he had amazed me even more in those weeks with his patience and kindness and courage. In him, Matthew had a constant, tender guardian, always making sure he was as comfortable and as well cared for as possible. No one could have done more.

———

Some days I would try to remember what my everyday life before the accident had felt like, by doing something ordinary, like wandering around

Leeds and trying to shop. One day, I decided to go out and attempt some Christmas shopping. I wanted things to be as normal as possible for Christian and Pippa. They needed some Christmas presents from their grandparents and I was determined to find some. I tried my best for a while before I sank exhausted on to a bench in the middle of Briggate and watched the people rushing around, wondering about their lives, the joys and sadness they must hold in their hearts. It was a year after the National Lottery had started and all I could see in my mind was the great big hand that had appeared in the television advertisements saying, 'It could be you.' In my imagination, it was pointing at me and saying, 'It *is* you' – not as a winner but chosen as a victim, and the tears started to roll uncontrollably down my cheeks.

Christmas came around and, despite all our dearest wishes, Matthew still hadn't woken up. He had been in his coma for two months. We didn't want him to be alone on Christmas Day, so Dena said she would stay with Matthew and we should go to Gaynel's in Manchester for lunch and try to forget our troubles for a few hours. The problem with Christmas is that it is such a sentimental time of year, when you tend to think back to other years and remember happier times, which made it all the more painful in a year when we were all so anxious and unsettled. We all made a big effort to keep our spirits up for Gaynel's two children, but we all knew what was lurking beneath the surface of the jollity for each of us.

As a special Christmas treat, Dena gave Matthew a taste of chocolate on his tongue. That was the full extent of his participation in the Christmas spirit that year. To help pass the long day in the sterile atmosphere of the hospital, Dena had a drink herself, which was a rare occurrence for her. It went straight to her head and she ended up tripping over one of the trolleys that littered Matthew's ward. Luckily no one came in to catch her lurching about.

It was around Christmas time that Matthew's professor, Martin, rang to say he had passed his PhD. Our son, who could now not speak a word, or even open his eyes, was a Doctor of Astrophysics. There was supposed to be an oral test as well, like an interview, after the thesis had been evaluated, but Martin had managed to persuade the authorities that under the circumstances they should award the doctorate on the strength of the thesis and Matthew's performance throughout the course. It was kind of him to go to so much trouble to ensure that Matthew was treated fairly and not penalised for something he could now do nothing about. It would have been an even greater tragedy if he had failed to get the PhD that he had worked so long and so hard to achieve. I couldn't wait for him to wake up and discover he had passed.

Just thinking about it made my heart swell with pride, but at the same time I wanted to cry when I thought about what he might have gone on to achieve next if the accident had never happened. Maybe he would have ended up a professor. Perhaps he would have written ground-breaking books and won prizes for his work. Who knows what heights he would have soared to, or what kind of man he would have become. How different Matthew's world would have been then.

————

The longer Matthew stayed in the coma, the lower his chances of making a good recovery if he woke up, or so we were led to believe by the experts. Whereas once I had sat by the bed willing him to pass away, now I was urging him to come back to us as quickly as possible, before the damage was irreparable, if it wasn't already. The frustration of every day that dragged by without any progress was agonising. I would have given anything for the chance to see Matthew walk up onstage to receive his doctorate, just like all his friends, but that was beginning to seem like an impossible dream.

One of the pieces of advice that a doctor gave us when we asked how long Matthew's recovery was likely to take, if it happened at all, was not to think in terms of 'weeks and months' but in terms of 'months and years'. If I had to wait years I could cope with that, as long as I could see at least a little progress. But it was beginning to look as if he might never wake up at all. Despite all Keith's optimism and willpower, it was starting to seem as if the first doctor had been right when he painted the worst-case scenario for us. Perhaps, I thought, he was right to break it to us so early. Maybe it would have been wrong for him to hold out false hopes for us.

Although Keith was as worried as I was, he refused to believe that Matthew wasn't coming back to us, and I clung to the strength of his conviction like a drowning woman.

13

The Opening of an Eye

Three months after the accident that had sent Matthew into the dark, something momentous happened. We had a sign that at least part of Matthew's brain was returning to consciousness.

One morning, we went in to see him and Keith immediately noticed that something had changed. 'Look, Mavis – do you see that?' he said excitedly. 'Look what's happened!'

One eye had opened. It was just the tiniest of slits, and at first we couldn't be sure that it was open at all. But after staring at it for ages, we became convinced that the eye had indeed opened. It was impossible to tell if his brain was taking in anything his eye might be seeing, but at least it was a step forward.

When Gaynel and Dena visited, we showed it to them with an air of great triumph and they were as excited as we were. This was it, we all felt. This was the beginning of Matthew's long trek back to us. But, of course, even though we hoped that he'd be up in just a few days, nothing seemed to change. The little slit stayed just that – a barely perceptible gap between Matthew's lids.

Each day Keith would be at Matthew's bedside first thing in the morning and would check how it was progressing. Every now and then, it would seem as if the eye had opened up a tiny bit more, although he could never be sure that he wasn't imagining it. Even when the doctor had warned us that we should think in terms of years for Matthew's recovery, we had never realised how slow the rise from the coma could be. In our dreams, we had imagined that one day Matthew would just open his eyes and smile and our ordeal would be over, but we soon realised it was going to be a much longer haul than that. If we thought that this eye opening meant that the old Matthew would soon be back with us, we were very much mistaken.

Once the doctors saw a sign of life, they instigated some new routines for Matthew. The nurses began to get him up out of bed into a chair for at least a few hours of the day. He had to be strapped into the chair otherwise he would just fall forwards on to his knees on the floor, which happened once or twice when the nurses forgot to tie him in. It felt like another small step in the progress back towards a normal life to see Matthew out of bed for the first time since the accident.

'I swear he's watching me with that eye,' his Auntie Cath said, when she came in. We realised that the slit was growing enough so that it did seem as though his gaze was following us round the room. Matthew looked like a rather stern pirate with his long dark hair falling lankly on to his shoulders and his one watchful eye. There was no other expression or movement in his face, and we had no way of knowing if the eye was sending any messages back to his brain or not, but if it was they weren't eliciting any reactions.

Once we had got over our initial excitement, we realised that his eye might be open, but there was still no sign of Matthew coming back to us. If this was as far as his recovery went, he would still be no more than the cabbage the doctor had predicted. We went back to waiting and hoping.

———————

It was a young nurse at the hospital who told us that once they were sure they had stabilised him and done all they could, they would move him to a rehabilitation centre called Chapel Allerton Hospital, which was well known for dealing with people who've suffered strokes and head injuries. We knew we were lucky to have such a well-respected institution in the area and I felt very excited at the prospect of Matthew receiving all that extra help and support.

'And then there will be another move on after that,' she continued.

'Aren't we lucky?' I said, wondering what other facilities there were to help people like Matthew recover from their problems. I was feeling guilty for all the times I had got cross and impatient with the staff.

'Well, after that you put him in a home some-where in the country,' she said. 'And then you can visit him occasionally, and get on with your own lives.'

'You get out of here,' I snapped, all my goodwill towards her evaporating in a second. 'Keith, I'm going for a ciggy. I don't want her in this room when I get back.'

She had brought back the words of the first doctor who had told us Matthew would never change, words that I had been trying unsuccess-fully to push to the back of my mind ever since. Following Keith's lead, I had decided that Matthew was going to wake up and start to get better. I refused to allow these people to decide arbitrarily that this was the best that Matthew could expect for the rest of his life. If we started to think like that, we might as well give up and go home like they suggested, and then he would be left to the mercy of whoever was being paid to care for him. The idea was unthinkable. We had seen the way that some of the professionals looked after patients who weren't in a position to speak up for themselves, and we suspected that a home where visitors only popped in twice a year was likely to be a hundred times worse than the busy, respected hospitals we had experienced so far. Putting him into a home would mean giving up all hope and we could never allow ourselves to do that, not with Matthew depending on us to protect him.

The poor little nurse was obviously shocked to see how deeply her words had cut me. She just stood there, looking stunned as I stormed out heading for a corridor I had discovered, where they allowed people to smoke without going outside. I lit myself a cigarette with shaking hands. That was someone else who wasn't going to like me much now.

Everyone kept telling Keith and me that we had to give ourselves a break from our vigil. In the end we gave in to the pressure and we agreed to go to Blackpool with a couple of friends. But only once we were sure there would be other friends and family popping in and out of the hospital all the time we were away. In Blackpool we tried our very hardest to forget about Matthew for a while and relax, but it was impossible. In the end we had to leave our friends on the promenade and go back to our hotel room together for a cry. Neither of us could bear to be parted from him for long.

Matthew's lung had mended at last and his breathing was growing easier so they took the tracheotomy tube out of his throat, and this in turn made swallowing simpler and less dangerous. We were then able to give him a few things by mouth, like drinks and soups, although he was still getting most of his nutrition through the tube going into his stomach. Having the tube to his throat removed was a big boost to our morale; breathing normally for himself was the first skill that Matthew had regained since the accident, and he looked so much better without that sinister-looking tube going into him.

———————

In the new year he left Leeds Infirmary and we all moved to Chapel Allerton, feeling optimistic that now we would be receiving more attentive, experienced and specialised care.

'Right,' Keith said, on the day of the move. 'This

is a chance for us to start with a clean slate. We're not going to argue with anyone and we are going to do whatever they tell us. We are going to abide by their rules. We're not going to turn him or touch him or do anything unless they tell us to.'

Although anyone listening to us talking might think that I am the bossy one of the relationship, when Keith finally puts his foot down, that is pretty much the end of any argument. I heard what he was saying and determined to try my very hardest to keep my mouth shut and make life as easy as possible for him and for the staff. This was our chance to keep on everybody's good side and maintain a positive atmosphere.

Despite all our resolution, by the end of the first day our good intentions had gone by the board. Matthew was due to be turned but the staff kept promising to 'come in a minute', just as they had in the other hospitals.

'Get hold of him,' Keith growled to me, and we went back to our own regime of loving care and attention.

Keith was so much better at nursing than me, so much more patient and tender. He was also much more at ease with the other patients. There was one man who was crawling around the ward on his hands and knees, stark naked, like a wild animal. The staff kept scooping him up and taking him off to a side ward to put some clothes on him but he would always come back. I was frightened by the thought that Matthew might be the same if he came round and I was too embarrassed to know how to talk to the man beyond saying hello, but Keith never had any such problem. He could talk to everyone the same, whatever their problem, even if they were crawling around naked. As a result, people responded to him. If he saw a patient in another bed needing help lifting a spoon to his mouth, then he would go over and feed them without thinking anything about it. I was seeing him in a whole new light. It was like he had discovered a vocation. I had always known he was a kind, patient man, but I had never realised just how deep his reserves of kindness and patience ran. I felt very proud of him and humbled by my own shortcomings.

When the crawling man left to be taken into a home because he was too much for his mother to look after, she came over to talk to us.

'You're Keith, aren't you?' she asked. 'My son always talks about you, because you've been so kind to him.'

Kindness is probably the most needed and necessary thing in any hospital. They have all the latest machinery and drugs, but sometimes I wonder if what the patients really need is some old-fashioned 'tlc', tender loving care. We all need to be well fed, well rested and comfortable in order to thrive, particularly if we have been ill. It seems to me that hospitals aren't always the best places for that, with their terrible noises in the nights, harsh lights and harassed, overworked staff. They do their very best in the circumstances and even if I didn't like everything I saw, I appreciated their hard work and the difficult situations they had to work in. But I can't help thinking that smaller, quieter environments are better for patients who are convalescing over the long-term.

I was so grateful, though, that there was somewhere like Chapel Allerton for Matthew, and for the care he received there.

———————

For all the months since the accident, Keith and I had been living in a bubble of unrealistic optimism, punctuated by tearful descents into an over-whelming sadness every so often, until we pulled ourselves together once more. We had been concentrating almost all our thoughts and energies on Matthew, occasionally distracted by friends and relatives coming to visit, or by skirmishes with hospital staff. Now that his eye was open, and there was a real possibility that he might wake up, we were realising how massive the task ahead of us was. We were beginning to feel a panic growing in place of the anxiety. How would we cope with the future? Whatever happened seemed to be fraught with problems and grief.

One morning the hospital priest came to see us and told us to keep our hopes up.

'There is a boy here called Steve,' he said kindly, 'who's been with us for a year and this morning he smiled for the first time. So there is hope.'

He may have meant well but it didn't inspire me at all. You can get lost, I thought, if you think that's a cause for hope. Matthew's going to do better than that.

Then a man one bed away from Matthew woke up from his coma unable to remember even the alphabet and I felt a familiar sense of dread in my stomach.

'Why don't you go to a meeting with the other parents?' someone suggested to us when we voiced our fears one time. 'The organisation is called Headway and they meet downstairs every first Monday of the month.'

As we were both going to be there that evening anyway, we thought it was worth giving it a try. It was always nice to break the monotony of nursing Matthew with something different, and I liked the idea of meeting other people who would under-stand exactly what we were going through. When you have something that is occupying your mind to the exclusion of virtually everything else, it is very hard to make normal conversation with other people. They wanted to talk about the weather and we wanted to talk about Matthew; they wanted to talk about last night's telly or the latest football match and we wanted to talk about Matthew. There was a limit to how much we could bore other people with an obsession like ours, particularly when nothing much was changing and we were just going over and over the same subjects. But the people at this meeting would be in exactly the same position. We wanted to know about their experiences in the hope that we could learn from them, and they would want to know about ours.

When we got there, the room was full of parents, a couple of whom had brought their children with them. One of them was a twenty-year-old boy who was blind and the other was a very severely handicapped forty-year-old man, who had been in a biking accident. Keith and I sat quietly and listened to what everyone else had to say. Some of it was depressing, but it was still good to know that we weren't alone in our struggles, that there were thousands of people out there who were coping with the same things we were going to have to cope with.

One set of parents told us that when their son first woke up every single thing was a 'fridge' to him. If they pointed to a table and asked him what it was he would say 'fridge', and the same with a cup or a bed. So I prepared myself for that. Another warned that when their daughter woke up, she was massively oversexed, thinking about nothing else. That seemed more upsetting to me than the fridge story, but at least I was prepared now if that happened to Matthew. Another girl had been badly disfigured in her accident and hated the way she looked when she woke up, frightened that no one would ever fancy her again, but her boyfriend had still married her.

Another mother told me how she used to get her head-injured daughter to write everything down as she thought of it, knowing she would forget it soon afterwards because her short-term memory was completely gone.

'There's a book you can get,' someone told us, 'called *Head Injury*. That will definitely help.'

We came away from the meeting feeling more positive and less alone, even if the future still held some frightening unknowns. Matthew might not be the son we knew when he came back to us, and no one could predict who or what he might be instead. We could only wait and see.

In the meantime, we got hold of a copy of *Head Injury: A Practical Guide* by Trevor Powell. It was published in 1994, so it was quite a recent book, and once we read it from cover to cover, we wished that we had discovered it four months earlier. Every medical term was explained; every question we had ever asked was answered in a language we could easily understand. By taking some of the mystery out of the situation, the book helped to lessen much of the fear as well. It didn't try to kid us that what we were facing was going to be easy, but at least it helped us to understand what it was.

'If you go down to B&Q you can get books that tell you how to do everything from build a fence to plumb a sink in,' Gaynel said, when she saw it. 'Why weren't you given a book on how to handle a head injury on the first day that they realised Matthew was going to have problems?'

The book didn't say anything about cabbages and vegetables; it actually said that people with injuries like Matthew's could get better. It felt like a weight lifting off my shoulders. Although I had become determined to back Keith up in whatever he was intending to do to help Matthew to recover, I had never been able to shake off the sound of that doctor's words and the terrible future he had predicted for Matthew. All the time we were fighting to get him the best care possible, I was wondering if it was a hopeless cause, and whether we were just another set of deluded parents who couldn't bear to face the truth of their son's condition. But this book told us we were right to keep trying, to keep fighting, because there was always a hope of breakthrough.

Those meetings and that book helped us more than any of the doctors or nurses or specialists. I wish I could send every family affected by the tragedy of a head injury a copy of *Head Injuries*. Although you hear about all the people who are killed in great disasters, and sometimes see the survivors who have lost limbs, you seldom hear about the people who came out of hospital months later with head injuries that would change their lives, and the lives of their families, for ever. I think families need help when their loved ones are badly injured in such a way that they will never be the same again. They've suffered a terrible loss that will last the rest of their lives, and they need treatment for their emotional injuries, just as surely as if they would for physical wounds.

Everyone needs to be told that whatever the doctors or the other experts say to them, they should always trust their own instincts and should always do things their own way. Of course it's always good to listen to anything anyone is willing to tell you and to learn what you can, but never believe that the experts know all the answers, or that your son or daughter won't have a different outcome to the one predicted. I know that now, but at the time I was still racked by uncertainty as to whether we were being unrealistic in our hopes for giving Matthew back at least part of the life he had once had.

14

The Awakening

One morning in February, four months after Matthew's fall, I went into the hospital while Keith parked the car and Bob, a patient in the bed opposite who had a brain tumour, called out a greeting.

'Morning, Mavis,' he said. 'Your Matthew spoke last night.'

'Did he, Bob?' I said, thinking that Bob must be going downhill faster than I had realised. 'What did he say?'

'I asked him, "Who was that visiting you?" And he said, "Auntie Cath."'

I felt a lurch in my stomach. How would Bob have known that Matthew had an Auntie Cath? Maybe it was true. Maybe Matthew had spoken.

Hardly daring to breathe, I went over to his bed. 'Hello, Matt,' I said.

'Hello,' he replied in a small, slurred voice. Both of his eyes were open. He was awake.

I couldn't believe it – at last Matthew had come back to us! He wasn't a cabbage, just as we had always known he wouldn't be; he was talking. He had recognised me and he had spoken. From a start like that, surely he could achieve anything. In the normal course of events I would have been horrified by the strangulated sound of his voice and the amount of effort it obviously took him to get out even one word. But when you have been half expecting never to be able to communicate with your son again, even the one word, 'hello', is enough to drive you delirious with relief.

Keith and I were both overjoyed. It is hard to put into words how delighted we were to see our son back from his lonely journey. I was so overwhelmed I think I probably went a bit funny that morning. I couldn't stop fussing him. I was stroking him and cuddling him, like he had just come back from a long trip, like I was welcoming him back from the dead, which in a way I was. Keith sat back and watched me with a wry smile on his face. He didn't seem quite as overwhelmed as I was, for the simple reason that he'd never believed that Matthew wouldn't wake up. He was just hugely relieved that the moment was here at last.

'You,' Matthew said eventually, sounding like ET. 'Go home!'

I was cut to the quick. I managed to stumble out into the corridor before I burst into tears. After all we had been through in the previous months I couldn't believe he could be so unkind to me. I had cried much less over the previous few weeks, all my energies going into keeping a tight control over myself, bursting out in anger more often than tears, but in that corridor all the emotion of the morning swept me away.

Then I stopped, and pulled myself together. What was I thinking of? Matthew didn't know what had been going on since October! All he knew was that he had woken up in a hospital confused and in a lot of discomfort, and his mother was fussing over him in a way she never normally did. I had got on his nerves, just as I might have done in the old days when I tried to boss him around, or asked him too many questions about his private life, or told him too often how great he was. He had reacted just as he would have done before the accident. Why was I crying at the first sign my son had come back to me? He was still the same old Matthew — how lovely was that?

I pulled myself together and went back into the ward, sitting quietly beside the bed, not fussing him any more, letting Keith do the talking, and just basking in the wonderful realisation that my son was awake and with me once more, albeit in a confused state with his limbs twisted and his voice distorted.

He was back. Even if he never got any better than he was at that moment, at least we knew his brain was working. Even if he couldn't walk or talk properly, at least he wasn't going to be a cabbage. And if there was even a small amount of recovery and understanding, it gave us something to latch on to and build on. While we hadn't been able to reach him at all there had been nowhere to start from, now at least we could communicate with him and begin to rebuild his physical skills, so perhaps he could comb his own hair or lift food to his mouth.

But while we were ecstatic that Matthew had woken up, we also knew that this was the start of the second leg of his journey back towards the man he had been before the accident. There was a lot of work to do.

It soon became clear that Matthew was not the same person he had been. Although he could talk, he was confused, and when we started to ask him about what had happened and what he remembered, it became clear that he remembered nothing at all. Not only had he forgotten the fall and everything that led up to it, he had forgotten the twenty-five years before that. He had forgotten his own past. He could recognise us, and his sisters and the rest of the family – but he had no memories of us or anything we'd ever done together.

This is not an uncommon effect of brain injury, but it was still a great blow to us. Would his memory come back? Was this just a temporary blip? As usual, the doctors were unable to tell us anything. Each injury is different — there is no telling what might or might not happen. They seemed to take Matthew's waking up very much in their stride, altering his routines and schedules to take account of his progress, but otherwise acting very much as if it was business as usual. I suppose that's what it was for them — they weren't going to be jumping about with joy in quite the same way as Matthew's family were when he woke up. I was desperate for more information but it seemed that there was nothing more to tell us. Like before, it was just a question of waiting and seeing.

But I hated the way Matthew had lost his previous life in this cruel way. It seems a peculiarly miserable fate to lose all knowledge of what your life has been. After all, who are we if we can't remember what we have done in the past?

That was the state in which Matthew had emerged from his long sleep and no one knew how long it would last.

Once the initial joy and excitement was over, we quickly got used to Matthew being back with us, and enjoyed his company again, especially as more of his speech and voice came back. Despite all the contortions of his body and his voice, I could still catch glimpses of the old Matthew, which gave me hope. To start with, there was the same twinkle in his eye whenever there was a pretty nurse around. For five months I had been very afraid I would never laugh again, but from the moment we re-established contact with Matthew the laughter started to flow. It wasn't that there weren't a lot of tears and frustrations and angry words as well, but at least we were talking with him again, rather than just talking at him. We were moving forwards, even if it was only an inch at a time.

When we realised that he had no memory of his life before the fall, someone visiting another of the patients in the ward suggested that we should tell him he didn't smoke and didn't drink, as he probably wouldn't remember that he'd done both those things. I could see what she was getting at, and it was probably a light-hearted comment, but it made me think. There was no way I was ever going to lie to my son or try to change him. If his memory was gone, I wanted to tell him everything that I knew about his past as soon as possible. But we were also quickly discovering that his short-term memory had deserted him too. He couldn't remember anything for longer than an hour or two and then it was as if it had never happened. So telling Matthew the truth or lies amounted to the same thing – he would forget it almost at once.

Once Matthew was conscious, the staff encouraged us to get him into a wheelchair and push him outside for some fresh air. There were some French windows by his bed leading on to a paved area beside a little stream, with some seats where we could go for our cigarette breaks. A few days after Matthew came round Keith announced he was going out for a cigarette break and Matthew made a sign, fluttering the fingers of his good hand on his lips, indicating that he wanted a cigarette too. That part of his memory was still there, or maybe it was just the addiction or craving for nicotine that was talking. He even knew, when Keith first put a cigarette in his mouth the wrong way, that he needed to turn it round. He didn't smoke as much as us, nowhere near, but now and again he would ask to

come out with one or other of us on our breaks.
I suppose most parents would prefer it if their children didn't smoke, but the health hazards associ-
ated with smoking seemed pretty unimportant
compared to everything else that was going on in
his life.

He remembered he was a vegetarian as well.
Besides remembering who he was and recognising
us, which was a relief because one of the other
patients had come round while we were there and
had asked for his mother, who had been dead for
a year, Matthew also recognised friends when they
came to see him. But he could remember nothing
about the good times he had enjoyed with them in
the past, or anything about their lives. One of them
told him he had just got a job in London.

'How much is the salary?' Matthew wanted to
know.

'That's the Matthew we recognise,' his friend
laughed. 'That's just the sort of question he would
always have come straight out with.'

What he couldn't remember was events. He knew
he had been to university, but he couldn't remember
being there. He knew we were his parents, and Dena

and Gaynel were his sisters, but he could remember nothing about being a child.

'It's like the difference between recognition and recollection,' is how he explained it to me later. 'It's like if the police ask you to describe someone who has mugged you and you can't conjure up the face of your attacker well enough to describe it to them. But if they called in some suspects and put them in a line-up you would recognise the face. I can recognise people, but I can't recollect how I know them or where I met them.'

To be without any recollections means you are unable to daydream in the same way as other people, you have to live every moment in the present, having no past to draw on and no way to imagine how the future might be. Because trying to remember was such an effort, it wasn't long before he stopped bothering even to make an effort. He just let life slide past him in a never-ending stream of consciousness, like an endless parade passing by in front of his eyes. He had no idea how the parade came to be there or where the people would be going once they had vanished from sight, but that didn't stop him from joining in the celebration as it happened.

There are some good side effects of having no memory, of course. Imagine being able to have a row with someone, knowing they will remember nothing about it a few minutes later. It gives you great freedom to say exactly what is on your mind, something I had always been rather prone to doing anyway.

We told him about his PhD, although he could remember nothing about the course or the many hours he must have spent writing his thesis, and asked him if he would like Martin Barstow to send his certificate to him.

'No,' he said, struggling with the words and emotions. 'I want to go and get it myself. I want it to be presented to me by the Lord Chancellor.'

My heart lifted to hear him voicing an ambition like that. As long as he had things he wanted to do and to achieve, then he would be struggling to make himself better. It would be all too easy to give up on the daily struggle of regaining control of his body and mind, and to just allow everyone else to take care of everything for him. I know I would have been tempted by that option. But he was showing that he intended to make a fight of it.

His voice had also changed. Now it was laboured and strained and as hard for other people to understand as it was for him to get the words out. By the time he had worked out the necessary muscle movements to form the words, he had often forgotten what he wanted to say, or the person he was talking to had grown embarrassed on his behalf and had finished his sentence for him. Even those of us who spent a lot of time with him sometimes found it hard to understand what he was saying. Keith would blame his own middle-aged hearing for not being able to pick up some of the words clearly. We would ask Matthew to repeat things, but by the time he had it was often too late and he couldn't remember what it was he was trying to say.

But the most joyous thing was that his sense of humour had survived, even though his laugh now came out as a strange hybrid somewhere between a wheeze and a bray, sounding like it almost hurt him to produce it. His good nature and patience also remained intact, apparently untainted by bitterness over what had happened to him. If we had been proud of him before, we were even more proud of him now as we saw him struggling to join in the conversations going on around him, and responding to the affectionate teasing of his friends and relatives.

We were always looking for new ways to pass the long tedious hours in the hospital. We discovered that Matthew was able to remember how to play noughts and crosses. It would sometimes take a long time for him to persuade his hand to make a mark in the correct square, but it was worth the wait, especially when he started to beat us. There were pathways opening up in his brain, but who could say which ones they were or what they might lead to? Was this as far as he was going to get, or was this just the start of the breakthroughs?

We couldn't possibly know, but we were sure that the darkest days were now behind us. Our son was back. We could at last begin to look forward and make plans.

———

There were some wonderful facilities at Chapel Allerton, including a swimming pool and Keith was able to get into the water with Matthew and the physio several times a week. I felt we had been so lucky to be able to be there. The physios would spend several hours with Matthew every week, trying to coax his left arm and leg to uncurl so that he could stand and sit normally. He had always stood so upright as a young man, almost as if he was a soldier on parade, with his shoulders thrown back, and seeing him curled and hunched was frustrating. His brain, however, simply refused to send out the right signals and the muscles were shrinking with lack of use, making recovery harder with every day. Some weeks there didn't seem to be any progress at all, despite everyone's efforts.

As well as reawakening his muscles, the therapists were also working on the instructions that his brain was sending out, trying to open up the pathways that had become so blocked and impassable. An occupational therapist would work patiently with him, laying out puzzles in front of him that would have been too simple for a five-year-old, encouraging him to stretch out for the right pieces and to coordinate his movements to achieve the desired results.

Everything that Matthew did was agonisingly slow and laboured and sometimes the frustrations would become too much for him to bear and he would let out a little bleat of anger or pain. Sometimes he would seem to be deliberately uncooperative as they tried to get him to instruct his feet to kick a balloon back and forth between them. There were always such long time delays with everything he was asked to do as the instructions tried to make their way to the right places and make his flailing limbs do as they were told. It must have often felt unbearable for Matthew, whose mind had once been so quick and agile, to have to struggle so hard to make even the simplest movement.

So many of the judgements we make about people are guided by their body language and their facial expressions. Even though both Matthew's eyes were open now, making him look more normal, he still didn't have full control of the messages his face was sending out. If a face remains unmoving and sullen, the head down and the body hunched and twisted, its owner appears to be a different person. It's easy to see evidence of this in the ways people react to anyone disabled. Those who didn't know Matthew would cock their heads on one side when they said hello, as if talking to a child, and then immediately turn their attention to Keith or me or whoever else was with him. Maybe they were embarrassed, not sure how to react to him, or worried they wouldn't understand what he was saying to them. But the physios and therapists were trained to see through what was on the surface to the lovely person still trapped inside. Sometimes even they would talk to him a bit like they were teachers with a small child, which would make him frustrated or even a bit angry, but they always seemed to understand how he must feel and never let his behaviour worry them.

Not all the nurses were quite as understanding of their patients.

'If I'd gone through what he's going through, I'd be angry too,' one registrar said when a nurse complained that Matthew had been bad-tempered that day, and I was filled with gratitude to him for not only understanding but for speaking up for Matthew.

Mind you, there was plenty to annoy us as well. Talking to one of the doctors about what Matthew was like before the accident, I proudly told him that Matthew had a PhD in astrophysics. Usually when

I said that to people they would say something about how sad it was for someone with such a good brain to have suffered such an injury, or make a comment about so much potential being rendered so helpless by one foolish mistake. All meaningless phrases, of course, but comforting to hear nonetheless.

'He hasn't actually received it yet,' the doctor grunted.

He was right of course, and I suppose I was boasting a bit, but it seemed strange that he should feel the need to puncture my pride like that, as if poor Matthew was getting above himself in some way when I suggested that he might be on the same intellectual level as the doctors. I didn't need any reminding of just how low Matthew's chances of ever excelling at anything again were. I just needed some kind words of encouragement.

There were times when Matthew could misbehave. He never wanted to take the tablets they gave him, and used to flick them across the room, so we had to start crushing them in jam, to fool him into taking them. But I liked that he did this because it showed he still had a mind of his own, even if it had been damaged, that he wasn't willing simply to allow other people to decide what he should and shouldn't do with his life.

Every little sign of a returning personality lifted my spirits. One day they asked him to write Keith's name on a blackboard. He did as they asked, clumsily and laboriously, quite different to the man who just a few months ago had written an entire thesis on astrophysics, but when he finished the name he added a full stop. It was a tiny gesture but one that he didn't have to do and it touched me. We had been scared that he would have forgotten the entire alphabet like the other man in his ward, but he had even remembered his punctuation.

Another big step was Matthew learning to feed himself again. The day that they took the feeding tube out of his stomach was a good one. At first, eating was very hard for Matthew. The process of swallowing was a difficult one that required a lot of effort and concentration but right from the start he obviously enjoyed it, and was a tidy and able eater. He started to put weight back on as well, which made him look a great deal more healthy. Feeding himself seemed like a big advance for Matthew, and another bit of progress towards a more normal life.

The biggest lesson we had learned over the previous months was that doctors didn't always know best. In our experience, it had often been the opposite. One father of another patient, seeing Keith patiently trying to get Matthew up on to his feet for a few moments even though his left foot still curled and wouldn't go down below tiptoe, decided to do the same with his boy. It was the first time the boy had stood in over a year. His parents were so proud of him when he achieved it and his mother asked me to take a picture of them standing together. It was a lovely moment.

The next day the father told Keith he had been informed he wasn't allowed to do that again.

'They say it's not good for him,' he explained.

'Don't take any notice of them,' Keith said. 'You do what you think is right.'

How would this boy ever move forward if he didn't take some chances and push his boundaries? It may be that Keith was being irresponsible in suggesting the other father followed his own instincts, but I suspect not.

We were beginning to believe strongly that, even

if we lacked the medical education, we often knew what was best for our boy, which was not an attitude likely to make us any less unpopular with the staff. But we didn't care what they thought, we just wanted to make Matthew as well as we possibly could.

15

Moving About

In April, two months after he had woken up, the physios said they thought Matthew was ready to operate an electric wheelchair for himself. It was a massive step forward. Our boy, who just a few months before had been written off as a vegetable, was going to be able to move around the hospital independently of us. It was as big a milestone as his first words, another huge step forward in the road back to a normal life. At that stage he could still only just about hold his head up and he sat slumped to the side of the wheelchair like a sack of potatoes, unable to pull himself up straight.

'It may take him a while to learn how to operate it,' the nurses warned as they lifted him into the seat and showed him where the controls were, but the moment they stepped back he was off down the ward in an almost perfect straight line. Whatever part of his brain was needed to operate this machine, it was working fine.

Now that he was mobile he could get himself around the hospital for a change of scenery whenever he felt like it. He could even get to the canteen three floors up by riding in the lift. Going for a snack one day with Dena, he zoomed down the corridor and into the lift so fast that he had pressed the button for the canteen and the doors had closed before Dena was able to catch up. Not sure what to do next, she decided to wait where she was and watched as the lights told her the lift was on its way back for her. The doors opened again and Matthew was still sitting there. He gave a little nod to beckon her in, a mischievous smile on his face. Tiny moments like that took on immense proportions for us, making us laugh and giving us hope that things were going to get better because we were all working together now as a family, including Matthew himself.

In his sessions with the occupational therapist Matthew had to relearn some of the most basic life skills, like making himself a cup of tea. The first goal was to make him as independent of other people as possible. There are so many things we all do every day without even thinking about them, which become major operations once there has been a head injury. Within the first few minutes of most days, we all turn off alarm clocks, get out of bed, find our dressing gowns and slippers, use toilets, brush our teeth, have showers, make cups of tea, get dressed, turn on the radio or television, open curtains. All the time we are performing these routine tasks our minds are probably on other things, working out what we've got in the fridge for dinner that night, planning a day's work, scanning a newspaper, reading the mail and deciding what to do about letters that require a response. But for Matthew, virtually every one of those tiny tasks was beyond his capability without assistance from somebody else. There are so many organisational and coordination skills needed to live a normal life that we take for granted and never think about until they are lost. Even a natural reflex like swallowing his own saliva required thought and effort. But, even so, things could have been worse.

'There are some patients who come in here and can't even remember that you have to plug a kettle in at the wall and switch it on,' the therapist told Keith. 'But Matthew has still got those skills, so he's already in a better position than a lot of them.'

Imagine feeling grateful that your grown-up son can remember how to plug in a kettle, when just a few months before he had been writing a thesis on subjects we couldn't begin to understand, travelling to destinations we had never been to and acquiring skills we hadn't even known existed. But we were learning to count our blessings because we knew those little things were now the important things. Our main goal was to try to get Matthew back to a place where he could live and function on his own again in the world. He might never work as an astrophysicist, but at least he should be able to feed himself, make a drink and use the bathroom – the basic skills needed for leading a clean and civilised life. Matthew's future may have changed irrevocably, but we were determined that he would still enjoy the best future possible, making the most of his potential. It was obviously going to be a long hard struggle but that didn't mean we had any intention of giving up.

―――――

Chapel Allerton Hospital was good for Matthew in so many ways. Our experiences over the previous few months had taught us to be grateful for any extra little bits of care he received. Now that I had more time to think, I remembered that he had been complaining about a toothache the previous August. He couldn't remember, but I was willing to bet he hadn't done anything about it by the time of the accident in October, so I asked if he could see a dentist. The hospital arranged for one to come to his bed and find the hole that needed filling. It was an obvious thing to be able to do for a patient, but I still found it impressive. It felt like the world was starting to view him as a person again rather than just a medical condition.

The doctors had some predictions for us though. They said that there was probably a limit to what

Matthew would be able to achieve and that, despite his talking improving a little, he would never be able to take part in group discussions or conversations. One strand of conversation at a time would be all that he could manage. He would never be able to join in with group activities or empathise with other people. It was unlikely that his memory would return and the chances were that he would be self-obsessed, uninhibited and selfish. It was all very depressing – it didn't sound like our kind, cheerful Matthew at all.

But there was good news too. They told us there was a special unit at St Mary's Hospital – which had once been a maternity hospital and where I had given birth to Gaynel. Matthew could go there for two weeks but places were limited and he would only be able to go if he fulfilled their criteria. There he would get continuous physio and one-to-one attention for the whole fortnight. It sounded like an excellent opportunity so we went for an interview with Matthew in his wheelchair. It felt like we were holding out a begging bowl but we knew we had to go through with it if we wanted Matthew to get the benefit of the facilities at St Mary's.

When we went into the room where the interview was to be held, we were confronted by a panel of eight people sitting in a semicircle. It was their job to decide if Matthew was eligible. Facing them was a daunting experience. One doctor at the end of the line was staring at Matthew without saying anything.

'What the fuck are you looking at?' Matthew slurred, made unusually aggressive by the pressure of being under such intense scrutiny.

The man didn't apologise or explain but said nothing, just averted his stare down to the papers in front of him and never looked up or spoke again through the whole session. It didn't seem like a mature reaction from someone who was supposed to be making a professional assessment of a patient with a head injury. Apart from that, however, the conversation seemed to go well, with all of us agreeing how good it would be for Matthew to get more physio.

Despite the prediction that Matthew would not be able to participate in group discussions, he proved himself perfectly capable of following this one. Our boy, condemned to life as little more than a cabbage, just kept on proving them wrong.

'What do you want to do, Matthew, when you've finished your rehabilitation?' one of the doctors asked.

'When Matt's better,' I said, as Matthew struggled to find the words, 'he's hoping to go back to living in Leicester and continue his life where it was before it was interrupted.'

In our hearts we all knew this was unlikely ever to be possible, however optimistic we might be about his recovery, but it was a line we were all saying in order to keep Matthew's spirits up, and to give him something to aim for. In reality, even we could see that there was little chance he would ever be able to move away from Leeds and his family again. They then asked us to wait outside while they discussed our case. They called us back a few minutes later.

'We have decided it's not right for Matthew to come to St Mary's,' they informed us.

'Why?' I asked, puzzled and disappointed by this change of heart on their part. The interview had seemed to go so well after Matthew's initial outburst.

'Because he's going to be leaving Leeds authority

area and moving to Leicester,' the spokesman explained, 'and our brief is to concentrate our resources on people living in Leeds.'

If I had never mentioned Leicester, and had just said Matthew hoped to come back to live with us and restart his life, which was much more likely to be what would happen, their decision might well have gone the other way. But because I had talked as if Matthew might have a rosier future than he had, they weren't willing to fund him. I was furious at their short-sighted, parochial attitude.

Keith and I couldn't even bring ourselves to thank them for their time. We just stood up and pushed Matthew back out of the room. I couldn't believe that they were willing to deny Matthew treatment that he would so obviously benefit from, on such petty grounds. It was a huge disappointment, but there was nothing we could do about it. We would have to struggle on, relying on our own resources to help Matthew achieve the best life he could.

'Can we take him home for a visit?'

It was the question we kept asking the doctors.

It wasn't just for Matthew's sake. We thought a change of scene would be good for him but we were also tired of spending our days inside the sterile walls of hospitals, particularly Keith, who hadn't even had the breaks I had. But they were very reluctant to let him go, as if doubtful that normal citizens like us would be up to the challenge of protecting Matthew from the dangers of the real world.

'Maybe for half a day,' said a doctor eventually, towards the end of March. 'But be warned – he will probably be sick in the car because of the motion and his balance problems. You'll need to have a physio with you as well, and an occupational therapist to have a look at the house and see what obstacles there might be for Matthew. They'll be able to suggest what you can do to fix them.'

It had all seemed so simple – just a straightforward visit home – but of course it was much more complicated than that. Nevertheless, we were determined to do it, so it was all arranged and a taxi was booked that could take the wheelchair, as well as all of us. We told the driver that Matthew might be car sick, and we were all prepared with a bowl, just in case. The driver seemed to think that the best thing would be to get the journey over with as quickly as possible, so he was racing round corners like a madman and we could see that it was making Matthew really uncomfortable.

'Bloody slow down!' Keith kept shouting at him, becoming increasingly frustrated by the man's inability to understand the problem.

Matthew managed to hold on until we were out of the car before finally throwing up, which was a tremendous feat of self-control, I thought.

Six months after the accident, Matthew finally rolled back through our front door. It felt like another milestone had just gone past on our long journey back to how things had once been.

The occupational therapist had to admit the house was already almost perfect for someone with disabilities. The corridors, doorways and bathroom were all wide enough for him to get about in his wheelchair, and pretty much everything was within easy reach. The therapist offered to arrange to have bars put around the house at various strategic points to help Matthew to lift himself in and out of the chair and the bath, but we didn't think any of it was necessary. We had every intention of getting him out of the chair and walking properly as soon as possible, so we didn't want to make it too comfortable and easy for him to keep living as an invalid.

Having satisfied themselves that the house was safe for Matthew, the doctors started letting us take him home for whole days when he wasn't due for any physio, although they always insisted he should be back in the hospital by nine at night, in time for bed. I could see that they couldn't have beds lying empty for twenty-four hours at a time if there were people who needed them.

Having Matthew at home was wonderful. It was such a relief to be able to be on our own again as a little family unit, not having to worry about hospital rules or timetables or the disapproval of passing professionals. Keith felt he could relax and focus all his attention on Matthew. We began to see what the next stage of our journey might be like. As long as he had been unconscious in the hospital it had been hard to imagine how we would ever be able to cope with him in the house, but now that he was awake and we were actually doing it, it didn't seem so impossible. I remembered how panicked I'd felt when I imagined a future where we were caring for Matthew on our own, and how I'd clung on to the doctors and the hospital. But now, it had changed. We could see that it would be something we could do, that it wasn't the impossible task we'd envisaged. We could even see how it would be easier and more comfortable for us all to have Matthew at home.

After a month or so of going back and forth, Matthew started to be less keen to return to the hospital at nights, unable to see the point of going back if it was just to sleep, and often too tired from his day's exertions to be bothered with the journey. Keith gave in to his pleas and Matthew started sleeping in his own bed at home. After about a month of our doing this once or twice a week, the authorities at the hospital called us in and told us off, like teachers telling off truants at a boarding school.

The doctors were now beginning to talk about discharging Matthew and putting him into a home where he could live out the rest of his life.

'Oh no.' Keith was adamant. 'We're not agreeing to that. If he's going anywhere, he's going home with us. We've proved we can cope with him. We'd like you to discharge him to our care.'

'But he has nine physio sessions a week here,' the doctor reminded us. 'If I send him home, that'll drop to three.'

Once again, it felt like a negative response that did no one any good. There was no sense that here was a good solution to Matthew's problem that would free up resources and that all we had to do was work out how to give him the phsyio he needed. Instead, the attitude was that if our idea went against the established systems, then it wasn't worth considering. It felt as though we were children who were constantly being told 'No' by adults, no matter what it was we asked for.

We weren't alone in our disappointment with the way many of the medical professionals treated us. Another father of a head-injured boy put into words exactly what we were feeling.

'They want us to check our brains in at the door when we come in,' he said, 'and pick them up again on the way out.'

This father had come into the hospital one day and found the curtains drawn round his nineteen-year-old son's bed. When he asked why they had done that, the staff told him it was a punishment because the boy had thrown his knife across the room when his meal was served.

'But he can't hold a knife,' the father explained. 'He can't use his right hand at all. That's what he's trying to tell you; that's why he's getting frustrated.'

The idea of 'punishing' a head-injured boy for becoming angry seemed extraordinary to all of us.

Because I kept on speaking my mind, just as I had at Leicester and Leeds, the doctors and nurses didn't seem to want to talk to me if they could help it, and they didn't seem to want to talk to Dena or Gaynel either. I guess we were all too aggressive in our tone. They were more willing to talk to Keith, partly because he was better than us at not rubbing people up the wrong way, and partly because they all knew him better, since he was the one who was always in there, sitting with Matthew, playing cards with him, helping him to cope with all the things he was having to relearn, and getting him to the toilet in his wheelchair, so he didn't have to soil himself.

They were having a game of cards together one afternoon when a doctor came over.

'When you've finished your game,' he said cautiously, 'I'd like to have a word with you, Mr Marsh.'

'What's it about?' Keith asked.

'It's about Matthew.'

'If it's about Matt I'd rather you talked to us when all the family are here,' Keith said, 'because it concerns all of us, not just me.'

When the doctor talked to Keith and me together, it became clear that they were still trying to get us to put Matthew in a home. Perhaps they thought Keith would be more open to reason without me there, but they obviously didn't know how stubborn he could be. Just because he could be more diplomatic than the girls and me didn't mean he wasn't just as determined to do things his way.

When we finally got the message through to them that if Matthew couldn't stay in Chapel Allerton we were going to take him home, the doctor said that he had to see a psychiatrist from Leeds Infirmary before she would finally discharge him into our full-time care.

'I'm not taking him to see any psychiatrist,' Keith

grumbled, feeling annoyed that they felt so unsure we would be able to look after Matthew as well as he could be looked after in a home.

'I'll make you an appointment,' she bulldozed on, taking no notice of anything Keith was saying.

The appointment was made and since Keith remained adamant that he didn't want anything to do with it, Dena and I decided we would go as the family representatives. Keith sat outside in the corridor with Matthew while we went in, none of us feeling in a very cooperative mood.

'Let him do all the talking,' I muttered to Dena as we went in.

We sat down and all remained silent for as long as the man could bear. 'Well?' he said eventually.

'Well, what?' I asked, innocently.

'You wanted to see me.'

'We didn't want to see you. The doctor said we had to see you before Matthew could be signed out.'

'I would like Matthew to come to Leeds on my psychiatric ward for two weeks,' he said. 'So I can assess him.'

'What will you do with him exactly?' I asked.

'I'll see him once a day and assess him.'

'How long will you see him for?'

'Three minutes.'

'Will he get physio?'

'No,' he admitted, obviously irritated that we weren't simply accepting what he was telling us would happen. 'We wouldn't be able to do it on that ward.'

'What would he do for the other twenty-three hours and fifty-seven minutes of the day then?' I wanted to know.

'What do you mean?'

'Well, we don't want him to just sit around in a ward for another two weeks if he isn't being helped with physio.' It seemed to me that that would be a backward step rather than a forward one.

He blustered for a while and then, when he realised I wasn't going to change my tune, he turned on me. 'You've wasted my time!'

'I haven't wasted anyone's time. The doctor said we had to see you. I didn't want to see you. My husband's sat outside because he doesn't want to see you.'

'I'll tell you something, Mrs Marsh,' he snapped, 'you'll need me before I need you.'

With that he got up and stalked out.

There seemed to be no point in spending any more time in the hospital after that. We took Matthew home for the final time that July, nine months after the accident, and three times a week brought him back in for physio. From now on any progress he made was going to be up to us.

'I'll make up the difference by doing stuff with him myself,' Keith said defiantly that first evening home. 'I've watched them doing it often enough. I'll have him walking by Christmas.'

16

One Step at a Time

Once the three of us were back at home together permanently, Keith could really concentrate on trying to straighten out Matthew's left arm and leg, which were still uncomfortably curled up; it became his full-time job. The physio had warned him that if he forced them straight too violently, which would be possible to do physically, Matthew's brain would react against the movement and would pull them back up even more tightly as soon as Keith let go, having exactly the opposite effect to the one he was trying to achieve.

Every other day Keith would fill a hot bath and lift Matthew into the water. Even though he had put some weight on, Matthew was still quite light and so it was easy for Keith to lift him. I was still constantly nervous about him putting his back out, as I had no idea how I would cope with Matthew on my own if that happened.

The warmth of the water would relax Matthew's muscles and Keith would then put some light pressure on his knee or his elbow, talking to him all the time, encouraging him, pushing him on.

'Close your eyes, Matthew,' he would say, 'and concentrate on pulling that left knee.'

If I was in the house, I would sit and cry as I listened to Matthew's moans of pain from the bathroom. It must have been just as bad for Keith but he wouldn't let him off, and each time he did it he managed to get the joints to loosen up just a fraction more. The improvements were so marginal it was almost impossible to see them, but they were happening.

At night his leg would be strapped straight, so that his brain would grow used to it, and stop bothering to pull it up, and during the day he had to wear another brace round his waist, like an old-fashioned corset. It had Velcro fastenings to hold him tight and make him sit up straight, like he used to before the accident.

Keith was very good at sticking to the regime. I would have found it difficult to continue putting Matthew through so much discomfort — his pain would have pulled at my heartstrings too much and I would have preferred not to do it. Keith wouldn't waver though. He was adamant that we had to do everything we could to get Matthew as close to his old self as possible before it was too late and the pathways in his brain had blocked up for good and the muscles had permanently wasted away.

I had always admired my husband's willpower, and I knew all the children had inherited it from him, which made me hopeful that, between them, Matthew and Keith could achieve what they wanted. Matthew could be lazy, I knew that, but if Keith said it had to be done he would go along with it without too much complaint. He never really complained about anything that much, and never seemed to feel sorry for himself.

Sometimes it felt as though we were kidding ourselves that there was any improvement — and perhaps we were occasionally, if only to keep our spirits up — but there was no doubt that over the weeks and months the efforts started to pay off. Pathways in Matthew's brain must have been opening up, his muscles gradually relearning what they were supposed to do. Slowly, slowly, his spine began to straighten and his limbs uncurl. Keith could remember enough from PE classes at school when he was a boy to have a rough idea of how muscles functioned and how they could be worked on. It wasn't quite the same in Matthew's case because with most muscle development the philosophy of 'no pain, no gain' applies; here, it was the brain we were trying to retrain, rather than the muscles themselves. We needed to persuade his brain to allow his limbs to unravel again and obey the commands it was sending them, and the only way to do that was with gentle persistence.

We had been so thrilled when he was first able to operate the wheelchair, but now we wanted to get him out of it. It was too easy to rely on artificial aids and not bother trying to get him back on to his feet. Our goal was to have him walking around again on his own.

―――――――

In August 1996, ten months after the accident, the whole family went to Blackpool, including the grandchildren and Matthew. Most of the time, Matthew's spirits were good and he stayed calm and cheerful, just as he had always been. If there were occasional, and understandable, bursts of frustration and anger, for the most part he seemed remarkably lacking in bitterness. But over the past few months he had frequently said that what was happening to him was just a nightmare and that one day he knew he would wake up and discover he had been dreaming. When we got to the pleasure beach, he was in almost as high a state of excitement as the children and said he wanted to go on the 'Grand National' ride. Gaynel and Dena pushed him through the disabled entrance and one of the workers on the ride helped to strap him on. They set off and we waited for their return.

The ride finished but the seats that came back were empty. Keith and I looked at each other in horror.

'It's all right, love,' I was told when I enquired anxiously what had happened to my family. 'They finish on the other side. They'll have to go round again to get back here.'

The ride started up again and sure enough they eventually arrived back. Matthew was as white as a sheet.

'Now I know it's not a dream,' he said, as we all helped him back into his wheelchair.

———

We returned from Blackpool to the same gruelling regime of physiotherapy and Keith's endless, untiring patience as he pressed on. Every day he worked with Matthew, determined to get him out of his chair and on his feet. He was convinced that Matthew wouldn't be confined to this contraption for the rest of life — he was going to walk again, if Keith had to spend years in the attempt. As it was, it took many months of exercises and pers-everance. Matthew, obliging as ever, tried to please his father and carried on doing his best, even though day after day, it seemed as though there was no progress at all. Christmas came again, for the second time since the accident, and Matthew still wasn't quite on his feet. But Keith would keep going until he was.

Two months later, the triumphant day came. It was as exciting as the moment Matthew had taken his first steps as a toddler all those years before — perhaps even more so, because you always expect a baby to start walking eventually, whereas Matthew's ability to walk was in doubt. It certainly wasn't something the doctors had ever expected to happen. To our great delight, Matthew climbed up out of his chair, with the aid of two sticks, and shuffled his first few steps since the accident. He had been confined to a bed and then a chair for a year and a half. Now, at last, he was able to begin his journey back towards true independence.

Seeing him standing there grinning at me was a wonderful moment. It was his and Keith's triumph — and we were all absolutely delighted. The boy they had told us would be a vegetable was up and walking about.

Even so, it was no quick fix. Once again, I was reminded how slow and painful every scrap of progress would be. For weeks, Matthew needed both his sticks to help him move along at a snail's pace. Sometimes the effort needed to do it seemed more than it was worth. But Keith wouldn't let up, and one day Matthew could walk with only one stick. Then, a few weeks after that, he made his way through the house alone and unaided — unsteady but definitely walking. Well, you might call it lurching, really, because Matthew's balance wasn't quite established. Nevertheless, it was a triumph, and it was all down to Keith's patience and perseverance, as well as Matthew's hard work.

If Matthew had still been in hospital or in a home there would have been no way the staff would have had the time to spend with him that Keith put in. Once he had got him balanced on his feet, he would make him walk up and down the hall with him, over and over again, up and down, up and down, endlessly patient, endlessly firm.

I would hear Keith's voice, like a kindly sergeant major, 'left, right, left, right', for hours on end as they shuffled back and forth. Sometimes all I wanted was for him to shut up – the same phrase, over and over again, ringing through the bungalow nearly drove me mad.

I don't know how Keith managed it because he didn't have the escape route I had of going to the office each day. I was able to immerse myself in my work so thoroughly that I could sometimes forget for an hour or two what was going on back at the bungalow as the two of them worked away together. By forcing myself to concentrate, I was able to do my job well and received three promotions over the next few years, but it was my husband and son who were making the real progress.

For three years they worked on getting Matthew's walking back to normal, day in and day out. No hospital or home would have had the staff available to do that. I doubt if many staff would have had the patience to deal with someone who was moving forward at such a slow pace. They would have assumed much earlier that they had got Matthew as far as they could get him, that his quality of life was good enough, and they would then have equipped him with the mechanical aids he needed to operate his life from a wheelchair. But Keith didn't want that for Matthew, and he had the time and the willpower to put in as many years as were necessary. I would never have had that willpower.

I admired my husband's dedication to Matthew and I also admired Matthew himself – if I had been in his situation, I would have given up the struggle almost immediately, and been willing to sit in a chair and stare at a television screen for the rest of my life rather than put so much effort into such seemingly marginal improvements. Perhaps most people are like that, which is why the doctors never expected him to progress as far as he did. Maybe the long-term care homes are full of people whose relatives were like me and accepted things as they were, rather than kept on fighting for as long and hard as Keith did.

His efforts were relentless and he always refused to say, 'Not today, I can't be bothered,' or, 'Maybe Matthew deserves a break from all this.' He worked away, never letting an opportunity pass for Matthew to persevere with his recovery. I had my job to go to for a change of scene, but Keith was always with Matthew, seven days a week. Every Friday evening, however, he stuck to his old ritual of going down to the Conservative Club with his friends for a few drinks.

'Just watch your dad when he goes into the bathroom to get ready to go out,' I would say to Matthew each Friday. 'He'll go in looking old and tired and after a wash and brush-up, he'll come out transformed. It's like watching a contestant on *Stars in Their Eyes*.'

Keith would wonder what we were both laughing at when he came out, spruced up and ready for his night out, looking almost like the young Teddy boy I first fell in love with.

———

Keith brought an exercise bike into the house and Matthew started going on that for ten minutes at a time, building up other lost muscles. I decided to have a go on it once too, thinking it might help me to lose a bit of weight. Having got myself all dressed up in tracksuit bottoms and trainers, I sat on the saddle and had one push at the pedals before giving up. I'd spent more time getting dressed than I spent on the bike.

Eventually, all the patient work started to pay off. The doctor had warned us we had to think in terms of months and years and, for once, they were right. As the years went by, the improvements, which were almost imperceptible from week to week, began to build up. All of it improved Matthew's quality of life as he gradually went from someone hunched, bent and confined to a wheelchair, to a man who could walk unaided and upright, like normal.

One of the few positive things to come out of Matthew's loss of short-term memory was that he quickly forgot the tedium of these endless exercise sessions. A few hours after finishing one walk, Keith could convince him they needed to go for another because they hadn't done any that day. That way he got him to do at least twice as much exercise as he would have been willing to do if he could have remembered just how many boring hours he had already spent that day going up and down the hallway in tiny, shuffling steps, trying to relearn the muscle coordination needed for normal movement.

Matthew was always a bit lazy and prone to taking the easy options in life, as his professor had admitted to us when talking about his PhD, but he was also the most obliging of men, just as he had been an obliging child, always doing whatever he was asked with a good-natured smile. Whenever Keith asked him to do something he might sigh a little, possibly even roll his eyes, but he would do it with a good spirit. Sometimes he might not want to make the effort to come with us to a family gathering in another house, or even for a trip down to the pub, but if we used a touch of emotional blackmail and told him it would spoil our fun not to have him there, he would give a small smile and come along without further complaint.

Once Matthew's walking was good enough for him to go outside the house under his own power, Keith started to take him for walks around the local streets and parks. It was a big jump going from walking on even floors, with no wind to blow him off-course, no potholes to stumble into or kerbs to trip over. Even a relatively flat-looking piece of pavement can have a treacherous slope to it when you are unsure of your balance. But every day, whatever the weather, the two of them would be out there, arm in arm. To start with they would just go round the block, but gradually they did more and more, going out two or three times a day, walking two or three miles at a time. It was like my father taking Gaynel out when she was a baby, and they too were talking and laughing all the time.

Matthew's left leg was still prone to letting him down, especially if he tried to break into a run, which he started to do once he had mastered walking. His gait was still slightly awkward, but no worse than someone who might have suffered a leg injury and needed to learn to walk again.

Keith suggested going to the gym to work on Matthew's movements and muscles but, at first, Matthew had laughed at the idea.

'How can I?' he wanted to know. 'I can't do anything.'

But Keith was adamant and it wasn't long before Matthew began to see and feel the benefits himself. Rebuilding Matthew's body was a project they could share, an ambition they could work towards together, and because they were both such good and patient men, they were succeeding, even if it was at a snail's pace.

As well as working on his body and his muscles, Keith also wanted to do all he could to rebuild Matthew's mind. He couldn't sit down and discuss astrophysics with him, but he could play games like rummy and Matthew taught him how to play chess. He was keen to do anything that would force Matthew to use his brain, chipping away at the blocked pathways, trying to open them up or find alternative routes round them. They may not have played chess 100 per cent correctly, but Matthew could remember a lot of the rules and the moves, and Keith reasoned that the more he played the more it would all come back to him.

When they were playing a game of cards, Keith would get Matthew to sit cross-legged. While his brain was distracted with the problems of outwitting an opponent, his hips were splayed out and growing used to stretching into more normal positions. As long as he had been hunched in a wheelchair, or even an ordinary chair, he was not extending the stretch of his body. Keith had seen the physio pressing

Matthew's knee into her chest and pushing it to the side, trying to pull the tendons to lengthen them and allow his legs a more natural movement. All he had to do was work out new ways to get Matthew to use his body without triggering the wrong reactions in his brain.

When I came home from work Matthew would want to teach me how to play whatever game they had been playing, but often I wasn't in the mood. I didn't have Keith's patience or perseverance, especially after a busy day in the office. If Matthew had been living alone with me, he would have received very little of the stimulation Keith gave him — I didn't have the talent for it that Keith had, and my energy levels were much lower. I did agree to play Scrabble sometimes, although I never won a game because Matthew didn't seem to have lost any of the vocabulary he'd had before the accident. I suppose words must have been stored in a different part of his brain to memories of events.

Once Matthew was walking unaided, and was able to walk as easily outside as he could inside, it wasn't long before he was plucking up the courage to go out for walks on his own. We never knew what had happened during these outings because he would have forgotten once he got home, but sometimes they must have been pretty eventful. Once he returned covered in mud from head to foot, with no idea how it had happened. Such setbacks never bothered him — why would they when he couldn't remember them? We all have memories of moments when we said or did things that still make us cringe with embarrassment, but Matthew was spared that. Each day started with a clean slate.

As his independence grew he started coming down into town to meet me from work in the afternoons. I used to look forward to having his company for the journey home. He would get the bus and knew where he should get off. Sometimes, of course, he would get it wrong. I would receive a phone call telling me he had got on the wrong bus and was now on the other side of Leeds. Even though he never had any idea where he was in those situations, and had no idea how to retrace his steps, he was not frightened to ask for help, and people always seemed to be happy to give it, particularly bus drivers.

One day I booked Matthew into a photographer's studio in the centre of Leeds to have some portraits done. We arranged for him to catch a bus into the city centre and meet me outside the Alders store at the top of Briggate when I finished work. He was there on time and we went for a coffee and to do some shopping. It all felt so natural and normal. The session at the studio was so easy and relaxed that the photographer was surprised to find that Matthew was head-injured. The pictures turned out to be a lovely memento of a happy day. At times like that it was possible to forget for a while that our family was still living under a black cloud.

Matthew himself found his new life difficult to come to terms with at times. Although he never grumbled or complained, Keith and I knew that he was finding it hard to grow used to his new and limited horizons. After he had been home for about four years, we asked our doctor if Matthew could have a weekly session with a psychologist to try to help him come to terms with the accident. Keith took him along to the first session and the psychologist came out to meet them in the reception area.

'If I can,' he told Keith, 'I would like to talk to Matthew on his own.'

'The only problem with that,' Keith pointed out, 'is that he won't be able to remember any of the conversation when he comes out of your office, so I won't know anything about what you might be suggesting.'

But the man insisted that he would get a better picture if he had Matthew on his own, so Keith agreed, and waited outside as Matthew went in. Half an hour later the psychologist came back out.

'I've had a chat with Matthew,' he said, 'and asked him if he would like me to treat him, and he says no.'

'Well, he would say no,' Keith said. 'He thinks he's recovering on his own and doesn't need you. *I* know he needs someone to talk to, but *he* doesn't. He hasn't regained enough cognitive abilities to be able to make the right decisions on things like that. That's why I wanted to come in with him.'

'Well,' the psychologist said, in a tone that suggested the matter was now closed, 'Matthew will tell you all about our chat.'

But, just as Keith had predicted, Matthew had

forgotten he'd even been in there by the time they'd got to the end of the corridor.

From the time Matthew came home, we had been working on his speech, trying to make it easier for people to understand him. The speech therapist we were allocated showed us some throat exercises that would help him, but Matthew found them very diffi-cult and in the end didn't bother with them. There are so many muscles involved in talking, combined with the swallowing mechanisms, that it is an incredibly complicated operation for someone whose messages are being delayed and misrouted. The act of talking requires a lot of swallowing motions to get rid of saliva. If you have to think about each one in order not to choke, it is bound to slow your speech down. Matthew was continually having to clear his throat with loud rasping noises, which would startle people until they were used to his company.

He managed to get by with what he could do, and never seemed to be self-conscious about the way he sounded. He was always perfectly happy to walk up to a stranger in the street to ask for directions if he got lost, which happened a lot once he was able to leave the house on his own. He had always been a quietly spoken man, particularly when compared to Keith and me and the girls, much more tactful than the rest of us. We all tend to shout about things to get our points of view across, whereas he would always remain calm and reasonable. I know that our voices make us a little intimidating for some people, but no one ever found Matthew intimidating. He was always much better at charming people and making them feel safe and comfortable.

Sometimes I looked at him, amazed at the distance he'd travelled since he was lying in the hospital bed, his body locked and immobile and his brain deep in a coma.

I always used to tell him that he had an angel watching over him all his life. When I said it again to him, he replied, 'So where was he that night?'

'He just nipped out for a second,' I joked. 'Went absent without leave. AWOL of an angel.'

He might have been unlucky with his accident,

but in many other ways, Matthew was very lucky indeed.

———

As the years went by, Matthew and Keith developed regular habits: going to the gym together, the endless walks, going to the pub and playing billiards. Sometimes, when Keith had had a few beers, I wasn't sure which of them was propping up which as they rocked back home together down the road.

Although there were times when the slowness of Matthew's progress was heartbreaking for Keith, he was also finding enormous rewards in rekindling his relationship with his son. Not many parents get a second chance to get to know their children once they have grown up and left home. Given a choice, of course, we would rather Matthew had been able to go off and live the independent life he had wanted to lead when he went to university, but at a purely selfish level we could now enjoy Matthew's company in a way we never could have done if he had just been visiting us every few weeks or months. We discovered he had a wicked sense of humour we had previously only seen glimpses of, and we realised he had reserves of inner strength and goodness that made us proud of him. It was remarkable how cheerful he was.

When we were all down at the pub or at family gatherings, Matthew was always good company, always laughing, even when he became frustrated by his inability to communicate as fluently with other people as he had once been able to. His words were still hard to hear and it would sometimes take people a little while to tune in to what he was saying and, in the general noise of group conversation, his brain would often not move fast enough to allow him to keep up. He couldn't always find the words or enunciate them quickly enough to interrupt the flow of a conversation at the appropriate moment, so often his comments, which might be cleverer and funnier than anyone else's, would be drowned out in the general hubbub of noise as everyone tried to have their say and make their voices heard. It was not easy for him, but the doctor who had previously predicted that he would never be able to join in general conversations had badly underestimated Matthew's courage and determination.

Two years after passing his PhD, Matthew was finally able to go down to Leicester to receive his certificate. We all went with him, and he was walked up on to the stage by a friend of his called Jo, a charming young girl who steadied him up and down the steps. I was so proud of him for making the effort to do it, watching how he was not afraid to talk to anyone who came up to him, beaming at everyone, even though he could remember nothing about the course that had led to the doctorate, or the life he had lived while he was doing it. Keith and I came back to Leeds with the girls afterwards, but Matthew stopped with his friends for the night because a lot of them were still there, finishing their courses.

It was wonderful when his friends invited him to visit them. About three years after the accident, he went to spend a week in Sheffield with some friends called James and Louise. We took him to the bus station in Leeds to see him off safely, knowing James would be waiting at the other end when he arrived.

'Will you know when you've reached Sheffield?'

I asked Matthew as I fussed around.

He pointed up to the side of the station where the word LEEDS was written in large letters.

'When I see the word SHEFFIELD,' he said with a twinkle, 'I'll know I'm there.'

We both laughed and I felt relieved he was showing so much independence and keeping his sense of humour. We had equipped him with a mobile phone, which was a godsend. He immediately knew how to work it and was able to remember which button to press to get Keith or me, and we were always able to phone him if he got lost to find out where he was, that was if he knew, mind you.

James rang a couple of hours later to say Matthew was not at the bus stop when they got there and all my worries bubbled back to the surface. We should never have let him go on his own! How would we ever find him now? What if he forgot his name and address?

I gave James Matthew's mobile number and he rang back a bit later to say he had managed to get hold of him. Because James had been a bit late arriving at the station, Matthew had got a taxi to

James's old house. James immediately rushed round to the old address and found Matthew waiting patiently outside for him, quite confident that he would turn up sooner or later. It seemed he had lost none of his fearlessness about travelling.

On another occasion Keith and I were ten minutes late picking him up after he had been for a visit to Bristol to see his old girlfriend, Janet, and her boyfriend. He was nowhere in sight when we drew up and I felt a familiar rising of panic. When we phoned him we found he had managed to get himself on to a bus home to Middleton, assuming that we were not coming for him. I felt huge relief at moments like that, knowing that he was so resourceful and so unbothered when things went wrong.

Having discovered he could, Matthew made a number of trips to visit friends, going to Leicester four times to visit a girl called Gabrielle and her husband, and even down to London to visit another friend called Simon.

Once he was strong enough to travel, we started booking foreign holidays, so that we could give him some visual stimulation other than the four walls of the bungalow or the streets around our area. The first few days in a new location would always be an anxious time for Keith and me. We would have to keep an eye on where Matthew was all the time, as though he was a small child, fearful that if he wandered off in the wrong direction we would never get him back. Every time we lost sight of him we would get a feeling of sick panic in our stomachs as we forced ourselves to stay calm and try to think logically which direction he was likely to have gone in.

Although a lot of people shy away from talking to Matthew, and are sometimes unsure what to say to us in his presence, anxious they might upset us in some way, anyone who has had any experience with head-injured patients will always know what to say. The subject will even transcend language barriers, as we discovered when a Spanish cleaning lady started talking to us one year. She told us that her nephew had been head-injured.

'He never got better,' she told us in her broken English, 'and my sister, she died of a broken heart.'

I could understand exactly what she meant. Despite all the fantastic progress Matthew had made from those early days when they wrote him off as a cabbage, it still broke my heart every day to think how his life had been spoiled.

On our way to Spain one year we lost him at the airport in England. He had gone off to the toilet and just didn't reappear. When he finally got back he was still just able to remember what had happened.

'I got talking to this backpacker,' he told us, and we could imagine how easily he would have fallen into conversation with a stranger like that. 'I told him I had a problem and he said, "Haven't we all, mate?" He gave me this.'

Matthew held up a small pack of weed for us to see. Horrified, we managed to throw it away before anyone else saw it and we got into trouble. We laughed so much as we boarded the plane to think we should have found ourselves in such a ridiculous situation at our ages.

On another holiday Matthew was standing at the edge of the hotel pool in Turkey. 'I'm going to dive in,' he told me.

'Please don't,' I begged, terrified he would bang his head.

He took no notice and executed a perfect dive into the blue water.

'I just had to prove I still could,' he said as he pulled himself back out on to the hot paving.

He was always telling us that inside he felt no different to how he had always felt. Even though he couldn't run or walk or talk in the same way, and couldn't remember things, he still thought about life in the same way. So I could understand why he would want to prove to himself that he could still do at least some of the things he used to.

The following year we tried Center Parcs, which was a mistake. All the activities there were designed for the fit and able. Matthew still went on a lot of walks through the forests, but trying to play badminton and tennis just made him frustrated because his balance and coordination were so badly damaged.

_____

On New Year's Eve 1999 we persuaded Matthew to join us at our local club for the millennium celebrations. We had a wonderful time and so did Matthew. It was an evening of fun, laughter and optimism as we celebrated the beginning of the new century. The whole place was full of excitement and there was a young girl there who was all over Matthew, dragging him out to dance.

I watched him dancing and enjoying himself with a great feeling of happiness. Five years before, all of our lives had been transformed. On one dreadful day, I had seen my son close to death, hooked up to machines in an intensive care ward, with a miserable twilight existence predicted for him. Who would have thought that we would be here like this, laughing and celebrating? That he would be walking and dancing, talking to people and having a drink with them? Of course things were different to what they might have been but we would never know what the alternative future was. What we did have was our precious son, still with us and still enjoying life.

He wasn't a pale shadow of a human being kept alive by machines, or locked inside his own head without communication or physical ability to care for himself. He wasn't even wheelchair-bound. He was a fit and active young man.

'You know, Mum,' he laughed as he sat back

down with me for a breather, 'I'm actually doing something different, because I never used to dance before the accident.'

That night I walked home with a new spark of hope in my heart. We had all been blessed. We were all still together. That was all we needed.

17

Matthew's Mind

It is now over ten years since Matthew had his accident. He still lives at home with Keith and me, and will for as far into the future as we can see. It is a happy life in many ways, with its daily routines. We all enjoy each other's company and laugh together a lot.

But this story is not all about our triumph over the accident. There is still a deep grief and great sadness for us. I know both Keith and I have aged a lot in the recent years with the worry about Matthew's present and his future. I wish so much he could have a life again, and enjoy some lasting stimulation but I don't think it will be possible.

Nine years after the accident the hospital finally signed Matthew off, admitting that there was nothing more that they could do for him. Our experience of medical treatment had been mixed. On the one hand, Matthew had wonderful care from the first moment of his accident. He had the best treatment available, without a penny's cost to us, and the most skilled team of doctor's, nurses and physiotherapists looking after him. The hospitals were fantastic and the staff were often wonderful. But on the other hand, we couldn't help but feel let down. There had been no counselling and no explanations, and often very little encouragement. Right from the moment Matthew arrived in hospital, his future was decided without all the options being given to us. And the further away he moved from intensive care, the worse it got. Staff were too rushed and overworked to give him the care he needed – thank goodness Keith was on hand to do what they couldn't. Once he'd left hospital, there was no interest in his fate at all except for a twice-yearly assessment for the first couple of years. I couldn't understand why they didn't want to follow up Matthew's case in more detail, to see how a man predicted to live the rest of his life as a cabbage had made such an amazing recovery. Couldn't it help other people in the same position? Perhaps it could give hope to another family as they sat, heartbroken and grief-stricken at the bedside of a beloved child who had suffered a head injury. Perhaps it could change the prognosis of that person to something better than the life they foresaw for Matthew.

It may well be that things have changed since our experience. I do hope so. Otherwise it seems like a great waste.

———

Everyone is always very impressed with how far Matthew has come — and he *has* come a very long way — but living with him day to day, we know it isn't really far enough.

Once Matthew was physically almost back to where he had been before the accident, Keith and I wanted to make sure he was mentally stimulated in the same way. Although we could discuss almost anything with Matthew, we were never able to talk astrophysics to him. Matthew needed someone to get him reading again in the same way Keith had got him walking and moving, get him thinking and talking about the subject that had fascinated him for so many years. But reading is hard if you have a short-term memory problem. How can you follow the plot of a novel if you can't remember what you read yesterday, or even a few hours ago?

When all is said and done, Matthew is a grown man who had no choice but to come home to live with his semi-retired parents. Keith and I had been all set to spend the rest of our lives comfortably living the same life we had always lived, the same conversations, same friends, same interests. But Matthew didn't want to spend all his time with people twice his age. We liked different television programmes to him; we had different things we liked to talk about.

'I've spoiled what should have been your golden years,' Matthew said to us quite soon after he regained consciousness, and I thought that was so selfless and kind of him. We were equally worried that we were spoiling his chances of restoring his thinking abilities to the level they should have been reaching. Living with two ageing parents in a bungalow in Middleton is hardly life on the intellectual edge. We feared we were blocking his progress by not being clever enough. He tried to do it for himself from time to time, but when he did get out a book he would have to put a ruler under the line he was reading to help him to concentrate, and progress was so slow he quickly lost interest.

Dena suggested that he should learn a poem to help stimulate his mind. Obliging as ever, he did as she suggested, reading a poem by Tennyson every day for a week and by the end of the week he had it memorised, which was an incredible feat. But he didn't do it again and I think I should have been stronger about nagging him to keep it up.

He seemed able to store some of the most important information, like how to get home from a walk, but most things were too trivial for him to be able to raise the energy to try to remember them. He needed someone to keep on at him, badgering him to think different thoughts, imagine different things and work on trying to remember.

When he first became mobile and able to move freely from room to room in the bungalow he was pleased with himself.

'This is good,' he said. 'Now I can get some variety by looking at some different cracks in the wall.'

It is a problem that we still haven't solved. How do you consistently stimulate a mind that can't remember anything but is sharp in every other way? At one stage we tried taking him to a day centre to give us all a break from one another and to allow him to mix with some different faces. We left him there for a day, but he became hopelessly bored and the staff said the gym was too dangerous for him because he was doing too many things. It seemed they were saying we had been too successful in bringing him back to life, that he was now inappropriately lively and interested in his surroundings. He also tried going to a photography class, but it was too basic for him.

'Why do I need to go to a class to learn what I can read in the camera's instructions?' he asked when he got home, and it was hard not to agree.

We bought a computer sometime after Matthew came out of hospital and put up a desk in his bedroom. To begin with he went on it every day, contacting old friends by email. He made new friends too, getting in touch with a woman in

Canada whose husband had sustained a head injury from a fall and eventually left her after sixteen years of marriage. She and Matthew struck up a friendship over the Internet and she told him he had saved her life with his good advice and understanding. He seemed to be able to communicate better through the means of a keyboard, where there was no hurry to find the right words and no problems about being heard above other voices.

His friends from university stayed very loyal to him in the first few years, all of them offering their support, visiting him when they could, and writing to him. Several times they came up to Leeds in the early days to take him to picnics and pop concerts in Roundhay Park while he was still in a wheelchair, and then there had been the trips Matthew made by bus to visit them at their homes. But their lives inevitably became busier and fuller as they left university and started to get good jobs and fell into new relationships. They would email or write to Matthew about their lives with less and less frequency, and he would even forget even when they had contacted him. No one ever has as much time for the friends of their youth once they're out of university and working to make their way in the world.

It was different for our generation because we all stayed in the same area and went to the same places with the same people all our lives, but Matthew's friends were dispersing all over the world, starting relationships and families as well as pursuing their glittering careers. I think that was the hardest thing for him, realising they were all drifting away and not being in a position to replace them with new friends because he didn't work, or travel anywhere without us, or do any of the things that people of his age usually did. Every day he was alone in the house with Keith and me, and even if he went out he only really met our friends. In reality, after his years away, Matthew had really come back to Leeds as a stranger after his years away and creating a new circle of friends has been impossible for him.

About two years after Matthew left hospital, I tried to find some form of help for him. I researched the Internet, scoured telephone books and asked everyone I met in the medical world. When they had talked about putting Matthew in a home I had imagined there were places specially for the young and disabled, which he might be able to visit for certain activities, but I soon realised they were just talking about care homes that were really just for the elderly. If we had agreed to having him sent away they would simply have sent him anywhere where the staff were willing to take on a head-injured person, wherever it might be in the country. Hilda had an uncle in a home in Blackpool who she used to visit twice a year.

'There was a young man about Matthew's age in there,' she told me after one visit. 'He was sat on some kind of beanbag in the corner of the room, head to one side, just staring into space. That could have been Matthew if you hadn't done what you have for him.'

There was a centre called Yorath Homes in Leeds, built by Terry Yorath, the Leeds United footballer, after his young son died one day playing football in the garden. They offered six- to twelve-month courses for the rehabilitation of injured people, but it was too expensive and the waiting list was too long to hold out any real hope.

My persistence eventually seemed to pay off when one day we were offered a half-day visit by someone to take Matthew out and about, getting him used to travelling again on buses, or even just going for a coffee in the centre of Leeds. I jumped at the offer, thinking it would give Keith at least a few hours of spare time. For the first few visits I booked time off work to see what went on.

The young lady who arrived chatted happily about her work and her boyfriend and the afternoon passed pleasantly. The same happened on the second visit. On the third one Matthew asked if she would like to take him to the local shopping centre.

'Oh, not really,' she said, 'I've already been there this morning.'

'OK,' Matthew replied, as obliging as ever.

'No,' she relented reluctantly, maybe seeing the look of surprise on my face, 'if you want to we can.'

'It's OK,' he said. 'I've changed my mind.'

She then went on to tell him how lucky he was compared to the young man she was going to see after leaving us.

'He's in a terrible state,' she said, 'dribbling, unable to feed himself. His parents really look forward to my visits and help.'

I decided after that visit to cancel her and try to

find someone else, but I never managed it. No one was going to be as good and selfless towards Matthew as his dad.

———————

That was really the last attempt we made to get Matthew some mental stimulation. It grieves me very much that there is nothing we can do for him on that score. My father had always said to me, 'Educate your children, Mavis, because no one can take that off them.'

But now I can see that he was wrong. After just one critical mistake from Matthew, one slip on life's road, Fate has taken away everything he had learned and everything he would have learned once he had gone out into the world with his PhD.

In some ways, I believe now that a head injury you can't recover from is the worst thing that can happen to you. If a loved one has died, you can at least mourn for them. If they are seriously ill, you can put all your faith into modern medicine and hope for a cure. Even if Matthew had broken his back and been paralysed, he would still at least have been himself, with all his memories and education intact.

But a head injury is different. Matthew is condemned to a very cruel turn of life without recollections and that, to me, often seems like no life. His memories are gone forever: he cannot sit and daydream; he cannot think of his childhood and smile; he cannot remember his first love, or actually ever having made love. He has to live in the present moment, getting what he can from it before it disappears into the hole where his memory used to be.

In a way, it is similar to Alzheimer's. But, for the most part, that happens to the elderly, and the consolation is that the loved one does not know what is happening and has already lived a long life. To see Matthew enduring something like this from the age of only twenty-five, even having to repeat a short shopping list over and over again before he ventures out to the local shop is heartbreaking.

I spend many dark hours awake, when it feels as if the whole of the rest of the world is asleep, grieving over what has happened to my son. The only consolation is that he cannot remember what he has lost. At my lowest moments, I think about when Keith and I die and I wonder if, after a short while,

Matthew will even remember us. It is hard to see anything but a bleak future. It is impossible not to worry.

For the last couple of years, Keith's back trouble has been very bad and that has meant that he hasn't been able to help Matthew get out and about and exercise in the way he used to. Keith has always been the keystone of all of Matthew's progress and development, and without his energy, Matthew's improvements have reached a plateau. He doesn't go out as much as he used to, and he doesn't have the same spirit of adventure he had a few years back. It is easy to see that he got to where he is because of Keith's untiring efforts. Without his father around, Matthew will, I fear, slide back towards the life the doctors originally predicted for him. I hope we can find a way to stop that happening before it's too late.

One day I complimented Matthew on the way he managed to stay so cheerful, whatever life threw at him.

'I've never seen you cry since the accident,' I said.

'If I started to cry,' he told me, 'I'd drown.'

Epilogue

Family life as we had known it came to an end in October 1995, when Matthew had his accident. Since then, it has been an extraordinary journey of immense grief, intense hope and many moments of triumph. Matthew is so very far from the person we were told he would be.

We did what we needed to do. We brought Matthew back from a state close to death; we gave him back his ability to walk and talk and eat and care for himself; we made sure he lived with us, and not in a home far away from us, full of people whose futures had been written off.

Of course we didn't do it alone. We had the unstinting support and love of our friends and family, and many of Matthew's friends rallied round to do their bit as well.

I myself have learned a great deal over the last ten years. I have learned that kindness is one of the most important things in life. Kindness to others is the best thing you can offer them, and I try to remember that constantly. These days I think of other people and what they are bearing a lot more than I used to, when life went on along an even keel. I didn't realise then how many tragedies are happening every day, and how many families are suffering. Today, tomorrow, the next day . . . each brings about another accident, and another family is plunged into the grief and chaos of losing a loved one, whether through death or through severe injury. I'm so glad that there are people to help. I only wish that more could be done.

I have also learned what patience and dedication can achieve — before, I was used to things being in my control and happening when I wanted them to. Now I can see that the smallest, immeasurable steps can add up to a great journey, just as has happened to Matthew.

I have some very black days and of course the grief will never go away. Neither will my fears for the future. But, for the most part, we are happy and positive. Matthew has his independence. He can make himself cups of tea whenever he feels like it. Every morning he gets up and makes his own breakfast and washes up the dishes. He sets himself new goals from time to time. He continued to smoke, like both of us, until about eight years after the accident when he decided to give up, just to show that he could, and he hasn't had a cigarette since. I don't know that I will ever find the willpower to do that, particularly if I had as many empty hours in the day as he does.

I'm very proud of Matthew, and of his attitude. He didn't turn out the way that some of the doctors predicted — that selfish, self-obsessed person they warned us about has never appeared.

He is still as laid-back and good-natured as ever. As I see it, even with what he has to put up with, Matthew is better than most. I never see him as being less than what he was before. He is what he is, and I love him exactly that way.

When I say proudly, 'Matthew can do everything!' he'll make me laugh by saying something dry like, 'I can't do ballet dancing.' When I explain to people that Matthew can't remember his past or what has happened recently, he says crypt-ically, 'But who knows what's real and what isn't?'

That's Matthew all over. He does so well to not let things get him down. Keith and I love him so much. He has come on an amazing path. It is not one we would have wished for him, but it is what Fate decreed, and it could have been much, much worse. He lived a wonderful life, full of travel and friendship and contemplation of the great mysteries of the universe. Then, after one tiny slip, he returned from death's door, foiled the expectations of the doctors and came back to us.

I cannot imagine life without Matthew, the boy

whose life was shattered but who has been put back together again, with patience, kindness and inexhaustible love.

Sleepless Nights

It's midnight now — what do I do?
I just sit and think of you,
I dream of days that have gone before,
I think of days ahead and hope for more.
When you were young, then you grew tall;
You shocked us all when you had your fall.
I live in hope — what can I do?
Just sit at night and think of you.

When each day dawns and sadness comes,
I look around at what you've done;

Each day you surprise me with your strength,
Your peace of mind is your defence.
You look at me and say, 'What can I do?
I never meant to hurt anyone of you
I must carry on — it was meant to be.
Walk at my side, help and comfort me.'

Mavis Marsh, 2006